T0039128

CURRENT STATUS OF CHITOSAN ON DERMAL/TRANSDERMAL DRUG DELIVERY SYSTEMS

BIOCHEMISTRY RESEARCH TRENDS

Additional books in this series can be found on Nova's website
under the Series tab.

Additional E-books in this series can be found on Nova's website
under the E-book tab.

DERMATOLOGY - LABORATORY AND CLINICAL RESEARCH

Additional books in this series can be found on Nova's website
under the Series tab.

Additional E-books in this series can be found on Nova's website
under the E-book tab.

BIOCHEMISTRY RESEARCH TRENDS

CURRENT STATUS OF CHITOSAN ON DERMAL/TRANSDERMAL DRUG DELIVERY SYSTEMS

IPEK OZCAN
TANER SENYIGIT
EVREN HOMAN GOKCE
AND
OZGEN OZER

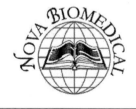

Nova Biomedical Books
New York

Library of Congress Cataloging-in-Publication Data
Current status of chitosan on dermal/transdermal drug delivery systems /
Ipek Ozcan ... [et al.].
    p. ; cm.
  Includes bibliographical references and index.
  ISBN 978-1-61761-298-5 (softcover)
  1. Chitosan--Biotechnology. 2. Transdermal medication. 3. Drug delivery
systems. I. Ozcan, Ipek.
  [DNLM: 1. Chitosan--administration & dosage. 2. Administration,
Cutaneous. 3. Drug Delivery Systems. QU 83]
  TP248.65.C55C87 2010
  615'.6--dc22
                                          2010031181

Published by Nova Science Publishers, Inc. † New York

Contents

Preface

In case of targeting the drug to the desired part of the skin, vehicles play an important role, beside the characteristics of the drug. Many natural and synthetic vehicles have been used for various topical dermal/transdermal preparations. However, chitosan has been standing out with its many advantages based mainly on its biological and physicochemical properties. Chitosan is a unique hydrophilic biopolymer obtained by partial deacetylation of chitin, which is one of the most abundant polysaccharide. It is a natural product widely found in crustacean shells, fungal cell walls, insect exosceletons, and mollusks. Chitosan is a linear glycosaminoglycan made up of N-acetyl-D-glucosamine units.

Characteristics of chitosan, such as the molecular weight, viscosity and the degree of deacetylation, greatly influence the properties of formulations. The by-products formed after the biodegradation of the polymer does not cause immune responses making it biocompatible. Due to the specific cationic glucosamine groups of chitosan, it can be interacted with anionic proteins in the skin providing the bioadhesive characteristics. These properties result in improved efficacy, enhanced bioavailability and reduced toxicity -generally recognized as safe (GRAS). Furthermore, the antimicrobial/ antibacterial and skin hydrating effects of chitosan have been received considerable attention for dermal/transdermal applications. It plays an important role in the cell regulation, tissue regeneration and collagen production. Chitosan and some of its complexes were approved by FDA for use in wound dressing products.

Chitosan also provides the controlled release of numerous active agents used for the treatment of skin diseases such as corticosteroids, antifungal agents, nonsteroidal anti-inflammatory drugs, hormones, local anesthetics, antiviral and antiseptic agents, etc. Regarding to the good bioadhesive property of chitosan and its ability to sustain the release of the active compounds, it has found many practices in the formulation of gels, dermal/transdermal patches, sponges, micro- and nanoparticulate systems as drug carriers. Particularly, chitosan has been used in the preparation of mucoadhesive formulations, for improving the dissolution rate of the poorly soluble drugs, drug targeting and enhancement of peptide absorption.

This paper is focused on the use of chitosan for dermal/ transdermal drug delivery systems following a general overview of chitosan. This natural polymer is a promising carrier or excipient as a delivery system and remarkable advances have been made about its potential applications in skin delivery.

Chapter I

Introduction

Skin is the largest body organ, weighing approximately 5 kg with a surface area of about two square meters in adult humans. This multilayered organ is an effective barrier protecting the body from the surrounding environment, thus being an efficient permeation obstacle for exogenous molecules [1]. When this barrier function is compromised for any reason, it becomes a port of entry for microorganisms into the body as seen in burns patients and various dermatological conditions [2].

The skin is composed of the outermost epidermis, and the dermis - vascular structure containing free nerve endings. The superficial layer of epidermis is the stratum corneum and it is almost impermeable and responsible for the barrier function of the skin. This highly hydrophobic layer is composed of differentiated non-nucleated cells, corneocytes, which are filled with keratins and embedded in the lipid domain. It plays a vital role in the absorption of drugs. Stratum corneum therefore, provides the rate-limiting step in the penetration process [3].

The penetration of drugs through the skin involves diffusion via *i)* transcellular pathways *ii)* intercellular pathways *iii)* hair follicles and sweat glands. The permeation through the appendages allows diffusional leakage into the epidermis and penetration directly into the dermis. This is supposedly the fastest route for hydrophilic molecules. However, the major transport pathway is through the intercellular lipid domains [1, 4].

Dermal (topical) delivery term is used to define a targeting within the skin, which involves ensuring minimal systemic absorption. This type of drug localization is important in the treatment of dermatological conditions such as skin cancer, psoriasis, eczema, and microbial infections, where the seat of the disease is located in the skin [5]. Dermal administration of drugs is performed for various destinations. Going from outside to inside the skin, the drug has to survive from the cleaning and protecting properties on the surface. Keratolytic and moisturizing effects, the stratum corneum and drug interactions with pharmacological targets localized in the viable epidermis and dermis are limiting factors for drug delivery. Systemic bioavailability is the aim of transdermal delivery [6].

Transdermal delivery is a term describing the situation in which a solute diffuses through the various layers of the skin and reaches the systemic circulation for a therapeutic effect [7, 8]. Transdermal drug delivery offers a number of potential advantages over conventional methods, such as pills and injections: *i)* no degradation due to stomach, intestine, or first pass of the liver, *ii)* probable improved patient compliance because of a user-friendly method, and *iii)* potential for controlled delivery. Nevertheless, very few drugs can be administered transdermally at therapeutic levels, due to the low permeability and lipophilic nature of human skin [6, 9].

To target the drug to the desired part of the skin, vehicles play an important role, beside the characteristics of the drug such as solubility, partition coefficient, particle size, charge and molecular weight etc. Many natural and synthetic vehicles have been used for various topical dermal/transdermal preparations. However, chitosan has been standing out with its many advantages based mainly on its biological and physicochemical properties [10].

Chitosan is a linear glycosaminoglycan made up of N-acetyl-D-glucosamine units derived from chitin by deacetylation. It is a natural product widely found in crustacean shells (crab, shrimp, crayfish), fungal cell walls, insect exosceletons, and molluscs. [11-13].

Since chitosan exhibits a variety of physicochemical and biological properties, it has found numerous applications in various fields such as environmental protection, agriculture, fabric and textiles, cosmetics, nutritional enhancement, and food processing [14].

In biomedical applications, chitosan and some of its complexes have been employed in wound dressings, drug delivery systems and space-filling implants [11]. Particularly, chitosan has been used in the preparation of mucoadhesive formulations [15, 16], for improving the dissolution rate of the poorly soluble drugs [17, 18], drug targeting [19] and enhancement of peptide absorption [10, 20, 21].

Chitosan has a very low toxicity and has been of GRAS status (generally recognized as safe) [15, 22], thus has found many practices in the formulation of gels, dermal/transdermal patches, micro- and nanoparticulate systems as drug carriers.

The aim of this chapter is to focus on the chitosan based formulations for dermal and transdermal applications by analyzing the physicochemical and biological properties of this natural polymer.

Chapter II

Physicochemical and Biological Properties of Chitosan

Chitosan can be produced in a variety of ways including thermal deacetylation, isolation from raw material and bioconversion methods [12]. Acetamide group of chitin can be converted into amino group to give chitosan, which is carried out by treating chitin with concentrated alkali solution [10]. Because of the presence of functional groups (amine and hydroxyl) various chemical chitosan derivatives have been synthesized and studied for different applications such as; thiolated chitosans, mono-N-carboxymethyl chitosan, quaternary chitosan and partially quaternized chitosan (N-trimethyl chitosan) [23].

Chitin and chitosan represent long-chain polymers having molecular mass up to several million Daltons [10]. Commercially available chitosan is in a range of molecular weights between 3800 and 20000 Daltons and has 66-95% degrees of deacetylation with different types of salts such as glutamate, hydrochloride and lactate [24]. Due to high molecular weight and a linear unbranched structure, chitosan is an excellent viscosity enhancing agent in an acidic environment. It behaves as a pseudoplastic material exhibiting a decrease in viscosity with increasing rates of shear [25].

The viscosity of chitosan solution is affected by its molecular weight, ionic strength, pH and temperature of solution. Low molecular weight chitosan oligomers provide a low solution viscosity [26]. The viscosity of chitosan solution is directly proportional to chitosan concentration and degree of deacetylation but inversely proportional to solution temperature and pH [25].

Chitosan with a low degree of deacetylation (of about 40%) is soluble up to pH 9.0, whereas with a high degree (of about 85%) is soluble only up to pH 6.5. Solubility is also greatly infuenced by the addition of salt to the solution. The higher is the ionic strength, the lower is the solubility [27].

The potential of chitosan stems from its cationic nature in neutral or basic pH conditions and high charge density in solution [28]. This polymer is distinct from other commonly available polysaccharides due to the presence of nitrogen in its molecular structure, its cationicity, and its capacity to form polyelectrolyte complexes. The cationic nature of the polymer allows it to become water-soluble after the formation of carboxylate salts, such as formate, acetate, lactate, malate, citrate, glyoxylate, pyruvate, glycolate, and ascorbate and show strong adhesive properties [29]. When adhesion is allowed to develop, substantial amounts of drug is delivered until a limit imposed by the drug partition coefficient [30, 31]. Adhesion to specific sites increases the bioavailability by optimum contact due to the extended time of residence [32, 33].

The mechanism of adhesion is predominantly explained by primary electrostatic interaction followed by secondary hydrogen bonding which is highly dependent on the ionic strength and chitosan possesses -OH and -NH$_2$ groups that can give rise to this confirmation [16, 34].

The strong mucoadhesive characteristic displayed by chitosan is the electrostatic interaction between the positively charged amino groups in chitosan and the negatively charged sialic acid residues present in mucins [28].

Chitosan salts as well as trimethylchitosan are able to enhance the paracellular permeability of intestinal, nasal and buccal mucosal epithelia by transiently opening the tight junctions, thereby increasing the paracellular absorption of hydrophilic and macromolecular drugs. In the last years it has been proven that tight junctions occur also on skin and have been characterised in the granular cell layer of human epidermis [35, 36]. The positive charge of chitosan salts and trimethyl chitosan might help them to be used as penetration enhancers due to the ionic interaction with negatively charged groups of glycocalyx [37, 38].

Chitosan and hydroxypropyl chitosan were found to be enzymatically degraded so that they can be used for biodegradable controlled-release dosage forms [12]. Chitosan breaks down slowly to harmless products (amino sugars), which are completely absorbed by the human body and these by-products do not cause allergic reactions/rejection and exert moderate immunostimulating effects [39, 40]. This attractive natural polysaccharide shares the benefits of other natural polymers (lysozomal degradation, etc.), but does not induce an immune response [29]. It is biocompatible with living tissues. In-vivo toxicity studies show chitosan to be inert, non-toxic and easily removable from the organism without causing concurrent side reactions. The LD50 (lethal dose 50%) of chitosan in mice was determined to be greater than 16 g kg^{-1} which is close to sugar or salt [10, 25].

Table 1. The summary of chitosan usage in dermal/ transdermal delivery systems

The role of chitosan	Aim	Formulation	Active agent	Reference number
Network Matrix Carrier system	Enhanced drug release and/or Skin absorption	Gels	Berberine	[65]
			Tiaprofenic acid	[66]
			Terbinafine HCl	[67]
			Nonivamide	[68]
			Propranolol HCl	[69]
			Clobetasol propionate and mometasone furoate	[70]
			Testosteron	[75]
		Patches	Nifedipine	[88]
		Sponges	Paracetamol	[93]
		Microparticles	Retinoic acid	[133]
		Nanoparticles	Aciclovir	[144]
			Gene-DNA	[149]
		Coated Liposomes	Cyproterone acetate	[156]
			17-β-estradiol, progesterone, cyproterone acetate and finasteride	[157]
			Aciclovir and minoxidil	[164]
			Lidocaine HCl	[176]
		Microneedles	Calcein and bovine serum albumine	[238]
	Controlled and/or Localized drug delivery	Gels	Fibroblast growth factor	[74]
		Patches	Lidocaine hydrochloride	[83]
			Etoricoxib	[87]
			Paclitaxel	[89]
		Sponges	Curcumin	[94]
			Norfloxacin	[95]
		Microparticles	Diltiazem hydrochloride	[110]
			Fibroblast growth factor	[131]

Table 1. (Continued).

The role of chitosan	Aim	Formulation	Active agent	Reference number
			Artocarpin	[132]
		Nanoparticles	Gene-RNA	[136]
			Clobetasol propionate	[137]
			Retinol	[145]
			Prolidase	[146]
			Gene-DNA	[150]
		Coated Liposomes	Oligonucleotide	[151]
			Quinacrine	[152]
			Glycolic acid	[161]
			Superoxide dismutase	[183]
	Wound healing and/or Improved regeneration and re-epithelization	Gels	No drug incorporated	[43]
			Fibroblast growth factor	[74]
		Patches	Silver sulfadiazine	[85]
		Sponges	Fibroblast growth factor	[96]
		Microparticles	Fucoidan	[106]
			Ampicillin	[130]

Chitosan's monomeric unit, *N*-acetylglucosamine, occurs in hyaluronic acid, an extracelular macromolecule that is important in wound repair [41]. There are two stages of dermal healing; the inflammatory phase and the new tissue formation phase. During the inflammatory phase, infiltrating neutrophils aid in the removal of foreign agents in the area. When the new tissue is formed, fibroplasia begins by the formation of granulation tissue within the wound space. It was found that chitin and chitosan could accelerate the infiltration of inflammatory cells, consequently accelerating wound cleaning. Therefore chitosan has been used as a wound dressing for proliferation and activation of inflammatory cells in granulation tissue [42, 43].

The *N*-acetylglucosamine moiety in chitosan is structurally similar to glycosaminoglycans (GAGs), heparin and chondroitin sulphate beside hyaluronic acid. These compounds hold the specific interactions with various growth factors, receptors and adhesion proteins. Therefore, the analogous structure in chitosan aid to exert similar bioactivity and biocompatibility [44, 45].

Chitosan inhibits the growth of bacteria and this effect is reported to be dependent on the molecular weight [46]. The variety of chitosan salts markedly inhibited the growth of most bacteria tested. Their inhibitory effects differed with molecular weight and the particular bacterium. It was shown that chitosan had stronger bactericidal effects for gram-positive bacteria than gram-negative bacteria [47].

Not only due to its multitude of applications but due to increasing environmental awareness, the ecological production of chitosan with its low cost makes this natural polymer superior to other synthetic compounds [48].

In view of the above-mentioned properties, chitosan is extensively used in developing drug delivery systems for dermal and transdermal applications. Table 1 represents the chitosan usage in various dermal/ transdermal delivery systems.

Chapter III

Chitosan Based Formulations

Gels

Gels are semi-solid dispersions of small or large molecules in an aqueous vehicle with a gelling agent. In other words, as stated by Peppas [49] they are macromolecular networks swollen in water or biological fluids. Gel formulations are suitable for topical delivery of drugs for treatment of diseases involving skin lesions due to lack of irritating components [50].

The development of hydrogels from a variety of synthetic materials has provided a great deal of flexibility in engineering the characteristics of the fabricated drug delivery systems. Polyethylene glycol (PEG), polyvinyl alcohol (PVA) and methacrylate derivatives have all been used to form hydrogels with variable mechanical strengths and biological responses [29]. However after many researches, chitosan gels were found to be advantageous and still preferable in comparison with other gel systems for dermal/transdermal drug delivery due to the favorable biological aspects. Especially its high capacity to adhere negatively charged membranes, causes enhanced muco/bioadhesion and improves wound and burn healing with low toxicity [25, 51, 52].

Hydrogels are often divided into three classes depending on the nature of their network, *i)* entangled networks, *ii)* covalently crosslinked networks and *iii)* networks formed by secondary interactions. However, with respect to chitosan hydrogels, this classification is not entirely suitable. Since the boundaries were not so district between these classes, a modified classification for chitosan hydrogels was offered as chemical and physical hydrogels. Chemical hydrogels are formed by irreversible covalent links, as in covalently crosslinked chitosan hydrogels. On the contrary, physical hydrogels are formed by various reversible links. These can be ionic interactions as in ionically crosslinked hydrogels and polyelectrolyte complexes, or secondary interactions as in chitosan/PVA complexed hydrogels, grafted chitosan hydrogels and entangled hydrogels [29, 49, 53-55].

The easiest way to prepare the chitosan gel is to solubilize chitosan in acidic aqueous media. The solubility of chitosan is the most crucial point for the preparation of gels. Chitosan is insoluble at alkaline and neutral pH values but is soluble in acidic media. The solubility of chitosan in acidic media is enhanced when its degree of deacetylation reaches 50% or more. In addition, the solubility of chitosan in inorganic acids is limited when compared with its solubility in common organic acids. Chitosan has a low solubility at physiological pH of 7.4 or higher pH as it is a weak base with pKa values ranging from 6.2 to 7 [56]. This type of chitosan hydrogels are limited by their lack of mechanical strength and tendency to dissolve. Moreover, they do not exhibit characteristics that allow drug delivery to be efficiently controlled [48].

Another way for the preparation of chitosan gel is the addition of covalent or ionic crosslinking agent [29, 48]. In crosslinked hydrogels, polymeric chains are interconnected by crosslinkers, leading to the formation of a 3D network. Crosslinkers are molecules of molecular weight much smaller than the molecular weight of the chains between two consecutive crosslinks. The properties of crosslinked hydrogels depend mainly on their crosslinking density; the ratio of moles of crosslinking agent to the moles of polymer repeating units [49].

The preparation of a hydrogel containing covalently crosslinked chitosan requires minimum amount of chitosan and crosslinker in an appropriate solvent, especially water. To date, the most common crosslinkers used with chitosan are dialdehydes such as glyoxal and in particular glutaraldehyde. However, the main disadvantage of these dialdehydes is that they are generally considered to be toxic [57]. Besides dialdehydes, epichlorohydrin, genipin, diioscyanate and oxalic acid are alternative crosslinkers. Among these alternatives, genipine is promising due to being naturally occurring and biocompatible [58]. Covalently crosslinked hydrogels are the only systems that are characterised by a permanent network, due to their irreversible chemical links. Therefore, they exhibit good mechanical properties and can overcome dissolution, even in extreme pH conditions [48].

In order to prepare ionically croslinked chitosan hydrogels, a charged ionic crosslinker and chitosan dispersed in a solvent (commonly water) are needed. Chitosan hydrogel could be obtained through treating the polymer with multivalent anions such as glycerol phosphate, oxalic acid, pyrophosphate, tripolyphosphate, tetrapolyphosphate, octapolyphosphate, and hexametaphosphate [56]. Ionic crosslinking is an extremely simple and mild procedure. In contrast to covalent crosslinking, no auxiliary molecules such as catalysts are required [59]. Ionically crosslinked chitosan hydrogels offer more possibilities as drug delivery systems compared to covalently crosslinked hydrogels. They can be formulated for controlled release not only in acidic but also in basic media and used for rapid release. However, their main disadvantages are the possible lack of mechanical stability and the risk of dissolution of the system, due to highly pH-sensitive swelling [48].

The pH of these systems has a substantial role in the swelling behaviour of chitosan gels. When pH decreases, the crosslinking decreases due to the reducement in crosslinker's charge density and swelling occurs. If the decrement in pH is too much, dissociation of ionic linkages and dissolution of the network can occur [59], leading to a fast drug release [60]. When pH increases the protonation of chitosan decreases and the crosslinking density declines thus blocks swelling. The protonation and repulsion of chitosan free ammonium groups helps swelling. If the pH becomes too high, amino groups of chitosan are neutralised and ionic crosslinking is inhibited. If the crosslinking density becomes too small, interactions are no longer strong enough to avoid dissolution and the ionic crosslinker is then released [61, 62].

An effective approach for developing a clinically applicable chitosan is to modify the surface of the material that has biofunctionality. Blending technologies with various additives may cause cytotoxicity. Hence, the modified biomedical-grade of chitosan with various derivatives must be submitted for biocompatibility testing [28, 63].

The technical properties and microbial stability of chitosan-EDTA were compared with well established gelatinizing agents such as carmellose sodium, hydroxypropylmethyl-cellulose, polycarbophil and carbopol 980. Chitosan-EDTA gels were shown to have the advantage of compatability with higher concentration of ethanol leading to excellent swelling and stability against microorganisms [37, 64].

Many drugs have been incorporated in chitosan gels in terms of dermal and transdermal drug delivery. The penetration of berberine into and through the rat skin was found in significant amounts after co-administration with absorption enhancers from chitosan gels [65]. Tiaprofenic acid loaded chitosan gel was compared to two types of emulsion (w/o and o/w) and hydrophilic petrolatum based ointment by means of *in vitro* release from cellophane membrane. The diffusion coefficient of the drug from chitosan gel was found to be the highest compared to all other vehicles [66].

In a study of Ozcan et al. [67], terbinafine hydrochloride loaded chitosan gels were prepared using different types of chitosan at different molecular weight, and the antifungal inhibitory activity was evaluated and compared to a marketed ointment product of the drug. Low molecular weight chitosan gel performed significant increament in antifungal activity caused by higher drug release resulting in larger zone of inhibition among other tested formulations prepared with medium and high molecular weight chitosan.

In vitro percutaneous absorption and *in vivo* pharmacodynamic responses of nonivamide (synthetic capsaicin) incorporated into chitosan, Pluronic F-127, carboxymethylcellulose gels and cream formulation were compared after topical administration to rats. Chitosan gels produced the highest nonivamide permeation across and the greatest cumulative amount trapped in the skin [68]. Propranolol hydrochloride was incorporated into physically cross-linked chitosan hydrogels with lauric, myristic, palmitic or stearic acid by freeze-drying for transdermal use [69]. The chitosan hydrogels provided more transcutaneous permeation of propranolol hydrochloride than the corresponding solution of the drug due to the possible enhancement of the drug solubility in the skin, probably produced by the interaction of the polymer with the stratum corneum.

Clobetasol propionate and mometasone furoate, as model drugs of topically applied corticosteroids, were loaded into medium molecular weight chitosan gels. Skin permeation was improved in comparison with commercial cream [70].

The release of cationic (lidocaine hydrochloride), anionic (benzoic acid) and neutral (hydrocortisone) model drug molecules from chitosan gel were studied for electrically-modulated drug delivery systems. The behavior of gels in an electric field resulted as changes in their surface pH during electrification and in the electrically modulated release of drug from the gel formulations. The results indicated that the release of the model drugs from the gel matrix was ranked in order as benzoic acid > hydrocortisone > lidocaine, which is consistent with the electrokinetically competing forces that are involved in these gels. Overall, effective and reliable electrically modulated drug delivery systems could be prepared using chitosan gels with adequate characterization of electrical effects on formulation matrices [71].

Taveira et al. [72] investigated the effect of iontophoresis on skin penetration of doxorubicin from chitosan gels. The results indicated that chitosan appeared to interact with negative charges in the skin. Hence, chitosan gel was reported to not only reduce electroosmotic flow, but also improve doxorubicin diffusion throughout the deeper layers of the skin.

In the area of wound healing, chitosan-based materials have been used in varying formulations. Chitosan itself can induce faster wound healing and produce smoother scarring [43, 73]. Chitosan hydrogels had an additional advantage for delivering a therapeutic agent to the local wound because of the reparative nature of the polymer. When chitosan hydrogels were tested as a carrier material for controlled release of fibroblast growth factor-2 (FGF-2) and as a wound healing acceleration property, a significant accelerated wound closure was observed and shortened healing process in mice [74].

Testosterone transdermal permeation enhancement from *N*-trimethyl chitosan gels with different degrees of quaternization were evaluated. Both *in vitro* and *in vivo* rabbit skin permeation studies suggested that transdermal permeation ascended with *N*-trimethyl chitosan formulations compared to the testosterone gel without enhancer [75].

Chitosan hydrogels have also been prepared as the carrier systems for a variety of different shapes, geometries, and formulations that include liquid gels, powders, beads, films, tablets, capsules, microspheres, microparticles, sponges, nanofibrils, textile fibers, and inorganic composites [29].

Patches/Films/Membranes

Patches are drug delivery systems intended for skin application in view of achieving local or systemic effect. In some cases, they might be of hydrocolloid characteristic and this helps them to serve as an occlusive and adhesive wafer dressing containing gel-forming agents. Patches provide the administration of effective and known drug amount to the skin [76].

The structure of the membrane depends mainly on the polymer type: such as molecular weight, deacetylation degree and also the polymer concentration in the film-forming solution [77, 78].

Lamination and casting techniques are well-known methods for the preparation of patch formulations and both of them could be implemented to the chitosan patches. Similar to gel formulations, solubilizing of chitosan in approriorate solvent is substantial for preparing patches. Lactic acid is generally preferred to solubilize chitosan because it has been proven to be non-irritating compared to other alternatives, such as acetic acid. Besides, lactic acid has the ability to improve the flexibility of the film due to a plasticizing action [79, 80]. Larena et al. [81] prepared several chitosan films using glycerine as a plasticizer alternatively.

Another important point for the preparation of chitosan patches is the choice of the chitosan type. In general, low molecular weight chitosan is preferable with greater patch properties such as being thin, transparent and less permeable to water vapor compared to patches prepared with high molecular weight chitosan [82].

A transdermal lidocaine hydrochloride chitosan patch was developed for rate control and a chitosan hydrogel as a drug reservoir. Drug release was found to be slower through chitosan membranes produced by a high degree of deacetylation with a larger thickness. The functionality of this transdermal patch was studied on the forearm of human volunteers. Patches prepared with a 95% degree of deacetylation, prolonged the anesthetic effect [83].

The degree of acetylation also plays a key role on some biological properties of chitosan gels. Chatelet et al. [84] demonstrated that the higher degree of deacetylation caused lower cell adhesion and proliferation.

The suitability of chitosan films (prepared with two different solvents: acetic acid and lactic acid) for wound dressing were investigated and compared with a commercial, polyurethane membrane supported gel, namely Omiderm®. In addition to physical characterizations (mechanical properties, *in vitro* bioadhesive strength and vapour permeability), the biological evaluations were also performed via primary skin irritation, intracutaneous and systemic injection tests. It was stated that chitosan films showed significantly better mechanical and bioadhesive strength properties from Omiderm®. Chitosan films prepared with lactic acid were found to be softer, more flexible and more bioadhesive than other tested films and did not cause erythema, edema or systemic toxicity [79]. Chitosan membrane loaded with silver sulfadiazine (AgSD) showed prolonged antibacterial activity and decreased potential silver toxicity as a result of the agar plate bacteria-cultures (*Pseudomonas aeruginosa* and *Staphylococcus aureus*) and cell-culture (3T3 fibroblasts) assays. The new formulation was less cytotoxic than the traditionally used AgSD cream, and was very effective for long-term inhibition of the growth of bacterium on an infected wound [85].

A series of chitosan based polyelectrolyte complexes were prepared in order to obtain films possessing the optimal functional properties (flexibility, resistance, water vapour transmission rate and bioadhesion) to be applied on the skin by the combination of chitosan and two polyacrylic acid polymers with different crosslinkers. The optimized film had shown appropriate properties for skin application and represented a promising formulation for further incorporation of drugs for topical and transdermal administration [86].

Etoricoxib transdermal patches were prepared using chitosan, its modified derivatives (with acetaldehyde and propioaldehyde) and chitosan-hydroxy propyl methyl cellulose (HPMC) blend with glycerol as plasticizer. The drug loaded films were cross-linked with sodium citrate and investigated for their permeation characteristics across dialysis membrane and rat skin. It has been observed that diffusion is the dominant mechanism for drug release following non-Fickian type of diffusion and the film prepared with acethaldehyde modified chitosan showed sustained release of drug [87].

Propranolol and nifedipin were evaluated for their transdermal delivery potentials using chitosan as a release controlling membrane. The membranes were permeable to both lipophilic and hydrophilic drugs. The drug release was significantly reduced when crosslinked chitosan membranes were used [88].

Drug-loaded chitosan films are emerging as alternative drug delivery systems and films appear to have potential for local sustained delivery of cancer chemotherapeutic agents such as paclitaxel [89].

Sponges

Sponges may be defined as dispersions of gas (usually air) in a solid matrix. There has been considerable recent interest in the use of sponges particularly as matrices for controlled drug delivery, as wound dressings and as matrices for cell growth within the tissue engineering field [90].

Sponges based on polysaccharides such as alginate and chitosan have been studied due to their low toxicity, favourable mechanical properties and capacity for bioresorption of the constituent materials [25, 91, 92].

As mentioned before the use of chitosan with different polymers is a general approach to modify the required properties of a formulation. The addition of alginate to chitosan were shown to accelarate the release of the drug (paracetamol) from the sponge. The use of chitosan and alginates together, was suggested as a strategy to manipulate both the mechanical properties and the drug release [93].

A biodegradable sponge, composed of chitosan and sodium alginate was investigated and it was seen that the gel's swelling ability was directly proportional to chitosan concentration in the sponge. The release of curcumin from the sponges have been extended for a period up to 20 days and could be controlled by the crosslinking degree [94]. In a similar study chitosan sponges including norfloxacin, the most effective parameter was found to be the degree of neutralization. It was also observed that the equilibrium swelling ratio decreased with increasing cross-linking density. The norfloxacin release was found to be swelling controlled initially and diffusion controlled at the extended release periods. It was also found that the antibacterial activity was directly proportional to the release rate [95].

Chitosan provided several advantages required for wound dressing. Wang et al. [96] assessed the biochemical and biophysical improvement of the chitosan crosslinked collagen sponge containing recombinant human fibroblast growth factor as a new wound dressing for the diabetic rats. The diabetic wound healing was found to be significantly improved by this formulation, as compared to collagen sponge alone and growth factor alone.

Particulate Systems

Chitosan has many advantages, particularly for developing micro/nanoparticles. These include: *i)* the ability to control the release of active agents, *ii)* avoiding the use of organic solvents in the preparation step since it is soluble in aqueous acidic solution, *iii)* the ability to crosslinking due to free amine groups, *iv)* easy ionic-crosslinking property with multivalent anions since cationic nature and *v)* increasing residual time at the site of absorption due to its mucoadhesive character [10].

Microparticles

Since the introduction of microcapsules by Green et al. in the 1950s, the term *microcapsule* is defined as a spherical particle with size varying from 50 nm to 2 mm and containing a core substance. The terms *microcapsules* and *microspheres* are often used synonymously and, *microbeads / beads* are used alternatively. *Spheres* and *spherical particles* indicates a large size and rigid morphology [73].

Microspheres are composed of artificial or natural polymers that can be modified to speed up or slow down the degradation of the polymer reservoirs (and, therefore, modify drug release kinetics) [97].

Chitosan-based particles can be prepared by both chemical and physical methods as listed; spray drying [98, 99], solvent evaporation [100], precipitation – chemical cross linking [20, 101], multiple emulsion method

[102], thermal cross-linking [103], complex coacervation [104], ionotropic gelation [105] and wet inversion [23, 62].

Reverse micellar and sieving methods has been suggested as new methods for preparation of micro- and nanoparticles of chitosan [10]. Supercritical fluid drying has been recently investigated as an alternative process for producing powder formulations. Critical properties of microcarriers have to be elaborated after the production by means of size and morphology, permeability, mechanical integrity, and biocompatibility [11].

Pharmaceutical applications of chitosan in the form of beads, microspheres and microcapsules were developed in the early of 1990's. Large chitosan microspheres and beads (up to thousands of microns) have typically been used for the prolonged release of drugs [106, 107] and proteins [20]. Small particle size (<5 μm) chitosan microspheres, containing anticancer agents such as 5-fluorouracil (5-FU) [104], and magnetic microspheres [108] have been described for site specific delivery. Cardiac agents [109, 110], anticancer drugs [111-114], anti-inflammatory drugs [115-120], steroidal drugs [20], antigens [121], insulin [122], growth factor [123], genes/DNA [26, 124, 125] and antibiotics [126-128] are the most studied groups for chitosan microspheres.

The strong interaction between chitosan microparticles and mucin was suggested to increase adsorption in biological surroundings by many studies [16, 100, 129].

The microsphere system based on polyion complexation of fucoidan with chitosan, was applied to treat dermal burns and the treatment period was shortened by improving regeneration and re-epithelization [106]. Similarly both of blank and ampicillin-loaded chitosan microspheres were shown to perform good wound healing properties *in vivo* [130].

Not only chitosan itself but also chitosan treated gelatin and alginate microspheres has found many applications in biomedical field. To provide a prolonged, site-specific delivery of basic fibroblast growth factor (bFGF) to the grafted skin in a convenient manner, biodegradable chitosan-gelatin microspheres were fabricated and incorporated into a porous chitosan-gelatin scaffold. The release kinetics of bFGF showed a fast release at the initial phase in the first 2 days, and the ultimate accumulated release was approximately 71.8% by day 14, indicating an extended time course for complete release [131]. In another study artocarpin (*Artocarpus incisus* extract) were loaded into alginate/chitosan microparticles for targeted transfollicular delivery. The efficiency of the loaded microparticles was shown to be comparable to the same dose of applied as solution. Moreover no systemic action was seen for microparticles as desired in a dermal application [132].

Chitosan treated alginate microparticles were prepared with the purpose of incorporating all-trans retinoic acid (ATRA) and microparticle characterization, drug–polymer interaction, release profiles and *in vitro* skin retention were investigated. The drug content of these microparticles was reported to be affected by ATRA concentration and by the solvent used and it was more weakly affected by chitosan concentration. The release of ATRA was also affected by chitosan concentration. *In vitro* retention studies indicated that maintenance of these microparticles in stratum corneum, improved the ATRA concentration in the deeper skin layers [133].

A transdermal drug delivery system of diltiazem hydrochloride was developed to obtain a prolonged controlled release with both matrix diffusion controlled and membrane permeation controlled systems. It was seen that zero order was fitted for the release of drug from membrane system, whereas non-Fickian pattern was fitted for matrix system. Membrane controlled delivery sustained the drug release more and exhibited a more steady state plasma concentration [110].

Nanoparticles

Polymeric nanoparticles are small colloidal particles which are made of non-biodegradable and biodegradable polymers with a diameter generally around 200 nm. These structures can enhance dermal uptake or improve tolerability of active substances and allow drug targeting to the different layers of skin [134, 135]. In the preparation stage, the choice of the polymeric material is a crucial step for developing pharmaceutical strategy. The percutaneous delivery of difficult-to-uptake substances might be facilitated by the selection of an appropriate polymer [134].

From a literature survey, it can be realized that the number of researches on chitosan nanoparticulate systems containing different active substances have been ascended due to its many advantages for developing nanoparticles.

Chitosan nanoparticles have been extensively investigated for site-specific drug and gene delivery systems. Chitosan nanoparticles as topical vehicles, have been proven to prolong the residence time and to sustain the release of active substance with respect to the skin [136, 137].

Considering the preparation method of chitosan particles, different techniques have been employed such as emulsion cross-linking [20], coacervation/precipitation [138], spray drying [139], emulsion-droplet coalesence [140], ionic gelation [141] and reverse micellar methods [10, 142, 143]. Screening of these methods depends upon several factors such as particle size requirement, stability of the active agent, stability of the final product and residual toxicity associated with the final product.

Many studies have been reported to assess the suitability of chitosan nanoparticles for dermal/transdermal drug delivery. The potential of chitosan-tripolyphosphate nanoparticles for delivery of aciclovir to skin was evaluated. The chitosan-tripolyphosphate nanoparticles loaded with aciclovir improved the chemical stability of the drug significantly and the permeation to skin was ameliorated especially from nanoparticles with higher chitosan content [144].

Beside the improvement in stability, the solubility of the drugs might also be increased by chitosan nanoparticles. The solubility of retinol was found to be more than 1600-fold by encapsulation into chitosan nanoparticles [145].

In case of dermal delivery, the challenge is the control of the drug localization in the desired layers of skin. Chitosan nanoparticles seem to facilitate the formulators to overcome this difficulty. Senyigit et al. [137] studied clobetasol propionate loaded lecithin/chitosan nanoparticles giving special attention to the transport across the skin by comparing the chitosan gel and commercially available cream of the drug. The accumulation in the epidermis was achieved without any significant permeation across the skin. In the light of this finding, a dose damping to 10% was offered for the reduction of the possible side effects of clobetasol propionate.

The potential toxicity of the applied nanoparticle is another serious matter to be dealt with for a researcher. Chitosan differs with its strong biocompatible nature among other polymers. Moreover longer and effective drug delivery can be obtained by these nanoparticles. Prolidase loaded chitosan nanoparticles suggested for prolidase deficiency (PD) were evaluated in terms of growth and the viability of cultured skin fibroblasts in order to verify the compatibility of the chitosan nanoparticles with cells. The results indicated good biocompatibility and further *ex vivo* experiments showed that prolidase loaded chitosan nanoparticles permitted to restore prolidase activity in PD fibroblasts for a prolonged period of time up to 8 days [146]. In another study the immunogenicity of antigen containing N-trimethyl chitosan nanoparticles were proved to induce dendritic cell maturation and to enhance immune responses [147].

Chitosan nanoparticles are shown to be good candidates for the delivery of DNA to skin. The topical application of chitosan-based nanoparticles containing plasmid DNA to the mice skin resulted in detectable levels of luciferase expression in skin after 24 h, and significant antigen-specific IgG titer expressed β-galactosidase 28 days after the first application [148]. Likewise, chitosan and poly-γ-glutamic nanoparticles for transdermal delivery were able to effectively retain the encapsulated DNA and also protect it from nuclease degradation. Nanoencapsulation improved penetration depth into the mouse skin and enhanced gene expression [149].

A multifunctional core-shell polymeric nanoparticles system composed of hydrophobic poly (D, L-lactic-co-glycolicacid) core and a positively-charged glycol chitosan shell were developed for transdermal DNA delivery and epidermal langerhans cells tracking. The core of the nanoparticles was used to load fluorescent quantum dots for ultrasensitive detection of langerhans cell migration following transdermal delivery. The results of animal studies indicated that bombardment of nanoparticles transfected DNA directly into langerhans cells present in the epidermis; the transfected langerhans cells then migrated and expressed the encoded gene products in the skin draining lymph nodes. This developed nanoparticle system would help to monitor and fine-tune important functional aspects of the immune system and thus offered as a potential for use in immunotherapy and vaccine development [150].

Ozbas-Turan et al. [151] prepared antisense oligonucleotide loaded chitosan nanoparticles and applied topically to rats for measurement of beta-galactosidase expression. The results indicated that free antisense oligonucleotides exhibited 35% of inhibition while nanoencapsulated antisense oligonucleotides inhibited approximately 82-85% of beta-galactosidase expression.

Liposomes

Liposomes are made from natural biodegradable and non-toxic phospholipid molecules which can entrap or bind different kinds of drugs into or on the lipid membrane [152, 153]. Numerous studies report that the application of liposomes on the skin surface is able to improve permeability for various entrapped drugs through the major barrier the stratum corneum [154-157]. As a result of liposome encapsulation, the drug was accumulated in the epidermis and dermis, therefore the systemic drug concentration was generally lower than that produced by the control preparations (ointment, cream, gel or lotion) [158]. Drug transfer mechanism from the liposomes is probably due to the similarity in the composition of the vesicle bilayer and the skin lipids, thus fusion of vesicles in the intercellular space of the skin occurs [159-161].

Liquid liposomes can be applied directly to skin. Generally it is impossible to incorporate liposomes in creams because of interactions between the surface active agents and the liposomal layers [162]. Due to the formation of a highly hydrated network of the hydrophilic polymers, liposomes are immobilized within the gel network and thus mechanically stabilized [163]. Hydrophilic polymers like chitosan are suitable thickening agents for topical application of liposomes in gel form. However, the type and concentration of the polymer, which forms the gel matrix, could influence the stability as well as the release rate of the incorporated drug.

The major drawback of liposomes is their instability during storage or in biological media, which is related to surface properties. They generally adhere to each other and after a certain time fuse to form larger vesicles. Biocompatible polymers have been used for the external surface modification of liposomes, obtaining a stable system for different way of applications [164-168]. Different types of biocompatible polymers such as chitosan can be employed to improve the efficiency of conventional liposomal systems [161, 169]. The biological properties of chitosan makes it a good candidate to combine to liposomes and to render them stable and bioadhesive structures [170]. Liposomes in a chitosan gel formulation can protect the encapsulated drugs against the degradation and provide their controlled and sustained release [171, 172]. Glavas-Dodov et al. prepared topical formulation by incorporation of liyophilized liposomes into the chitosan gel base. Liposomes embedded into a structured vehicle of chitosan gels sustained the release more than hydrogels [173, 174].

By combining the advantages of chitosan and liposomal characteristics, specific, prolonged, and controlled release may be achieved. Chitosan-coated liposomes were formed via ionic interaction between the positively charged chitosan and negatively charged diacetyl phosphate or phosphatidylcholine [175-179]. Several authors have used chitosan as a liposome coating to increase the stability of drug release [167, 169, 172, 180] and for targeting purposes [161, 177, 179, 181, 182].

Positively, neutrally and negatively charged liposomes were coated with two types of low and medium molecular weight chitosans. Both types of chitosan coating increased the mucoadhesive characteristics of all three types of vesicles. Using chitosan coating, high efficient superoxide dismutase-loaded vesicles for drug targeting on mucosal tissues could be produced [183].

Stability of aciclovir and minoxidil encapsulated liposomes and skin permeation were improved by coating with chitosan. The coating of liposomes led to higher skin diffusion for both drugs, which was explained as an effect of positively charged liposomes to interact stronger with skin's negatively charged surface and their possible interactions with structures below the stratum corneum. This interaction might result in transfering to deeper layers, disrupting the tight junctions in lower epidermis [164].

There are number of factors that can influence a polymer/colloid system such as chitosan/liposome ratio. A small change in one factor may seriously alter the stability as well as other characteristics of the system. Lidocaine hydrochloride chitosomes (liposome-chitosan combination) were prepared by coating multilamellar liposomes with chitosan to achieve an increment in the positive charge on the liposome surface. A high chitosan concentration was required at a low stirring range for production of the systems [176].

Ruel-Gariépy et al. [184] reported that negatively-charged liposomes were able to interact with thermosensitive chitosan hydrochloride (Protasan®) - based hydrogel to decrease slightly the gelation rate and the gel strength thus they could be useful for delivery of hydrophilic molecules.

By taking advantage of the biodegradable and biocompatible properties of chitosan, Chung et al. [152] developed the fibrin encapsulated liposome-in-chitosan matrix (FLCM) for sustained release of water soluble, low molecular weighed drugs. FLCM was offered for developing depot delivery system with a high volume capacity of reservoir.

Skin Tissue Engineering

Tissue engineering is a rapidly growing area that seeks to create, repair and/or replace tissues by using combinations of cells seeded on a scaffold, biomaterials, and/or biologically active molecules [185-187]. Skin tissue engineering offers exciting opportunities in the treatment of acute wounds (burn and skin excision), chronic wounds (diabetic ulcer, pressure ulcer), vitiligo and the scar revision surgery. Fibroblasts, the main component of dermal cells, can be easily isolated and cultured in monolayers by conventional cell culture techniques and they may enhance cellular motility in the wound. These cells play an important role in epithelial morphogenesis, keratinocyte adhesion, and the formation of the complex dermal-epithelial junction [188, 189]. The development of human skin models that have the same properties as genuine human skin is of particular significance [190, 191].

Protein-based polymers including collagen, gelatin, fibrin and other natural polymers such as alginate and chitosan are widely employed for tissue engineering. These polymers can provide not only physical support for tissue regeneration but also serves as biomimetic matrices with biological functions to actively induce tissue regeneration [192, 193].

The pioneers of skin tissue engineering focused on the application of collagen matrix as a cell carrier [194]. Similarly, chitosan was incorporated in tissue engineering because of its excellent biocompatibility and biodregadability. Chitosan could be easily formed into structures under mild processing conditions and chemically modified. Furthermore it has excellent wound healing properties as mentioned previously and an ability to be processed into porous structures for use in tissue regeneration [21, 195-201]. Table 2 summarizes applications and approaches of chitosan usage in dermal healing.

Physicochemical properties of chitosan influence fibroblast proliferation. Howling et al. compared the ability of 37, 58 and 89% deacetylated chitosan to modulate fibroblast mitogenesis *in vitro*. Results revealed that highly deacetylated chitosan was generally more capable of stimulating fibroblast mitogenesis [202].

In the inflammatory phase, chitosan has unique hemostatic properties that are independent of the normal clotting cascades [203]. The incorporation of collagen to chitosan was proven to enhance the cell attachement ability when compared to solely chitosan [204]. Because of the reasons cited above, a number of researchers have studied collagen-chitosan scaffolds as dermal equivalent in various tissue engineering applications [205-210]. Generally, composite scaffolds were prepared by freezing and lyophilizing of the collagen-chitosan solution. The effect of physical interaction between collagen and chitosan on biological properties of scaffolds was described by Tangsadthakun et al. [211]. The fibroblast proliferation was enhaced by chitosan containing scaffolds compared to pure collagen assayed by cell culture studies.

A skin equivalent based on a collagen-glycosaminoglycan-chitosan dermal substrate has been developed to meet the growing demand in tissue engineered skin equivalents [190]. Damour et al. [212] co-cultured fibroblasts and keratinocytes on a substrate composed of collagen-glycosaminoglycan-chitosan to treat a large skin defect. Skin resections were treated with a tissue-engineered graft with good wound regeneration. Further, the papers were published highlighting the clinical potential of this matrix and healing of dermal, epidermal lesion and burn [188, 213].

Table 2. Different applications and approaches
of chitosan usage in dermal healing

Aim	Formulation	Content of structure	Reference number
Wound healing	Wound dressing	Chitosan-fibroblast growth factor	[21]
		Chitosan-minocycline	[195]
		Chitosan-hyaluronic acid-chlorhexidine diacetate	[199]
		Chitosan-peptide	[201]
		Chitosan-plasenta	[222]
		Chitosan-fibrinojen	[222]
		Chitosan-collagen	[96], [205] [206], [208] [209], [210] [211], [214] [215]
		Chitosan-gelatine	[216], [218] [219], [220]
		Chitosan-glycosaminoglycan-collagen	[188], [190] [212], [213]
	Suture	Chitosan - poly (ε-caprolactone)	[232]
Hemostatic activity	Wound dressing	Chitosan-collagen	[204]
	Bandage	Chitosan acetate	[228]
	Suture	Chitosan-poly(L-lactic acid)	[235]
Antimicrobial activity	Bandage	Chitosan acetate	[229]

A biodegradable chitosan- nanosized collagen membrane as a novel skin substitute was developed and evaluated by animal studies. The membrane seeded with fibroblasts was found more effective than both gauze and commercial wound dressing, in healing wounds. An *in vivo* histological assessment indicated that covering the wound with the membrane resulted in its epithelialization and reconstruction [214]. Furthermore, the glutaraldehyde-treated collagen/chitosan scaffold was also pointed as a potential candidate for dermal equivalent with enhanced biostability and good biocompatibility [205, 215].

Chitosan-gelatin scaffolds have also been investigated for skin tissue engineering. Gelatin is a partially denatured derivative of the fibrous protein collagen and it can be completely resorbable *in vivo*. The chitosan-gelatin scaffolds were found more wettable than chitosan alone. The artificial skin obtained with chitosan-gelatin had suitable flexibility and mechanical properties for skin tissue engineering. Moreover the results indicated an inhibition of scar formation [216, 217]. Similarly, the researchers have proved that chitosan scaffolds containing basic fibroblast growth factor loaded gelatin microparticles were effective in accelerating wound closure of pressure ulcers [218]. To further enhance the properties of chitosan-gelatin scaffolds for skin tissue engineering, hyaluronic acid was introduced to chitosan-gelatin complex by Liu et al. to provide a new scaffold for skin tissue engineering [219, 220].

An increament in cell or DNA damage is associated with high toxicity therefore the newly developed chitosan derivative in the form of porous skin regenerating templates were tested for biocompatibility with human epidermal keratinocyte cultures and assessed in terms of cytotoxicity, genotoxicity and inflammation. Chitosan templates were found to be cytocompatible, non-toxic and capable of stimulating cell proliferation [221].

ChorioChit (Chorion/placenta + Chitosan) was offered as a biological wound dressing based on chitosan, combined with a human placenta extract. The dressing was found effective in the treatment of hard-healing wounds. ChitoFib (Chitosan + Fibrinogen) was another surgical biological dressing that combined the biopolymer chitosan and tissue glue developed on the basis of fibrinogen. The dressing enabled surgeons to replace wound stitches with glue [222].

Many of the chitosan based commercial product available in the market are basicly for wound healing as dressings and hemostatic products as patches, pads and granules (Table 3).

Cosmetic Applications

Chitosan is an excellent cosmetic excipient that is remarkably well tolerated by the skin. Since it is an efficient trapper of heavy metals that are responsible for many contact allergies; its usage in cosmetics may avoid skin allergies. Chitosan has a wide application as moisturizing component in different cosmetic investigations. Chitosan forms a protective tensor film on the skin's surface allowing active principles to be placed in close contact with the skin. Thus other hydrating agents, solar filters, organic acids or other active principles can be combined with chitosan to facilitate their effects [203, 223-226].

Therefore cosmetic compositions based upon chitosan is promising upon variety of applications for treatment of hair or skin. Moreover chitosan may be an essential component in cosmetics due to its antibacterial properties. Chitosan based products can be provided as hair care systems (hairspray, setting lotion, colouring products, shampoo), creams, lotions, cleansing products (cleansing milk, face peel, facial toner, soap) and as cosmetic agents for the care, protection, or cleaning of skin [227].

Table 3. Chitosan-based commercial products available in the market

Product	Formulation type	Medical application
Tegasorb®	Hydrocolloid dressing	Partial and full thickness dermal ulcers, superficial wounds, abrasions, burns
Tegaderm®	Transparent film dressing	Leg ulcers, sacral wounds, chronic wounds
Beschitin®	Patch	Dress burns and other wounds has an analgesic efect and favours early granulation, no retractive scar formation. For traumatic wounds, surgical tissue defects.
Syvek patch®	Patch	Hemostatic, achieving hemostasis.
Vulnosorb®	Sponge	Wound healing
Chitipack S®	Sponge like chitin	For traumatic wounds and surgical tissue defects. Favours early granulation, no retractive scar formation.
Chitopack C®	Cotton-like chitosan	Complete reconstruction of body tissue, re-building of normal subcutaneous tissue, and regular regeneration of skin.
Chitipack P®	Chitosan layer	For the treatment of large skin defects. Favours early granulation. Suitable for defects difficult to suture. After skin tumor surgery
HemCon Bandage®	Bandage	For emergency use to stop bleeding. Antibacterial, biocompatible wound dressing designed to be stuffed into a wound track to control moderate to severe bleeding.
Chitoseal®	Pad	Hemostatic in bleeding wounds
Clo-Sur®	Pad	Antimicrobial barrier, hemostatic wound dressing
Aquanova®	Pad	Leg ulcers, diabetic ulcers, surgical or traumatic wounds, minor and other burns, superficial cuts, lacerations and abrasions, and minor irritations of the skin.
Celox®	Granules	Emergency haemostat, minor cuts and bleeding
Chitodine®	Chitosan powder with adsorbed elementary iodine	For the disinfection and cleaning of wounded skin and for surgical dressing.
Chitopoly®	Chitosan and Polynosic Junlon poly(acrylate)	Antimicrobial wears, suitable to prevent dermatitis

Other Applications

Chitosan has found many applications in different tools such as bandage, suture and microneedle because of its versatility and beneficial physicochemical and biological properties.

Bandage

Chitosan's properties allow to rapidly clot blood, and has recently gained approval for use in bandages from FDA. Chitosan is hypoallergenic, and has natural anti-bacterial properties, further supporting its use in field bandages. Chitosan acetate bandage was developed as a hemostatic, antimicrobial topical dressing. This product performed superior properties when compared with gauze and alginate bandage [228]. Dai et al. [229] have demonstrated that the chitosan acetate bandage performed better than the clinically approved nanocrystalline silver bandage when it is topically applied to third-degree burns that are heavily contaminated with pathogenic bacteria.

Pads

Mechanical closure devices are not available to achieve fast and secure hemostasis. As an alternative chitosan pads were investigated and found to be useful for improvement in hemostasis. In a study, the use of chitosan pads significantly decreased the bleeding time in the first three minutes after manual compression time ($p < 0.01$) [230].

Suture

The application of chitosan fibers as sutures is remarkable due to its low immunogenicity [231]. The acceleration in wound healing and absorbtion by human body, favors its use since no second operation is required. It was reported that the chitin suture was absorbed in about 4 months in rat muscles. Moreover, application in patients proved satisfactory results in terms of tissue reaction and good healing. Toxicity tests, including acute toxicity, pyrogenicity, and mutagenicity were found negative [232]. It is known that successful wound healing depends on an appropriate tensile strength provided by the suture materials. In a study, with regard to wound healing in subcutaneous tissue, chitin administration significantly increased the tensile strength of skin sutures within 5 days, compared with the control [233].

Standard silk and catgut sutures coated with regenerated chitin or chitosan showed good wound-healing activities [234]. Chitosan coated poly(L-lactic acid) wires showed better hemostatic activity than wires without chitosan [235].

Microneedle

Transdermal drug delivery systems have been limited because of the strong barrier function of the skin. The use of micron-scale needles showed a dramatical increase of the skin permeability of drugs [236, 237]. It was suggested that the micro-needle patch of chitin and/or chitosan made insertion of the microneedles into a living body easier. Chitosan was pointed as a promising polymer for microneedle-mediated release of drugs through skin for enhancing transdermal drug delivery [238].

Future Directions

Drug delivery systems have changed to meet the needs in the area of dermal and transdermal therapy to obtain a sufficient efficacy with low toxicity. The demand for developing new formulations, coupled with the shortcomings of synthetic polymer based systems, caused the progress of less toxic and natural polymer based systems.

Numerous arrays of choices for these natural polymers as drug carriers are available, which offer different perspectives of formulation design.

As being a biocompatible, antimicrobial and cationic natural polymer, chitosan stands out for applications of dermal and transdermal drug delivery. The cabability of building up a matrix for different dosage forms such as hydrogel, patch, micro and nanoparticles and the ability of enhancing the adhesion properties of the formulations with its unique cationic charge, makes chitosan one of the first choice natural polymers.

The accelarated wound and burn healing observed with the chitosan added formulations or engineered skin tissues is another promising field in the area of dermal treatment.

As stated by many scientists, potential applications of chitosan in medicine can only be exploited if its usable forms are properly developed and prepared. Drug products for human use should be safe, efficacious and of an acceptable quality. Evidently, there is a lot to drive benefit from chitosan in dermal/transdermal treatments by these means. Interdisciplinary collaboration, especially the collaboration of clinicians with formulators would facilitate emphasizing the advantages and disadvantages of chitosan, to indicate where the future attempt should be set to. As such industry will be more willing to provide leadership in the area to further advance applications of the technology and the approval and marketing of chitosan based systems will ascend.

References

[1]   Godin, B and Touitou, E. Transdermal skin delivery: Predictions for humans from in vivo, ex vivo and animal models. *Advanced Drug Delivery Reviews*, 2007, 59, 1152-1161.

[2]   Bucks Daniel, AW and Maibach, HI, eds. *Topical absorption of dermatological products.* . Occlusion does not uniformly enhance penetration in vivo. 2002, Dekker: New York, NY. 9-32.

[3]   Barry, BW. Drug delivery routes in skin: a novel approach. *Advanced Drug Delivery Reviews*, 2002, 54 Suppl 1, S31-40.

[4]   Tadicherla, S and Berman, B. Percutaneous dermal drug delivery for local pain control. *Therapeutics and Clinical Risk Management*, 2006, 2, 99-113.

[5]   Brown, MB; Martin, GP; Jones, SA and Akomeah, FK. Dermal and transdermal drug delivery systems: current and future prospects. *Drug Delivery*, 2006, 13, 175-187.

[6]   Heuschkel, S; Wohlrab, J and Neubert, RHH. Dermal and transdermal targeting of dihydroavenanthramide D using enhancer molecules and novel microemulsions. *European Journal of Pharmaceutics and Biopharmaceutics*, 2009, 72, 552-560.

[7]   Naik, A; Kalia, YN and Guy, RH. Transdermal drug delivery: overcoming the skin's barrier function. *Pharmaceutical Science and Technology Today*, 2000, 3, 318-326.

[8]   Thomas, BJ and Finnin, BC. The transdermal revolution. *Drug Discovery Today*, 2004, 9, 697-703.

[9]   Prausnitz, MR and Langer, R. Transdermal drug delivery. *Nature Biotechnology*, 2008, 26, 1261-1268.

[10] Agnihotri, SA; Mallikarjuna, NN and Aminabhavi, TM. Recent advances on chitosan-based micro- and nanoparticles in drug delivery. *Journal of Controlled Release*, 2004, 100, 5-28.

[11] Hernández, RM; Orive, G; Murua, A and Pedraz, JL. Microcapsules and microcarriers for in situ cell delivery. *Advanced Drug Delivery Reviews*, In Press, doi: 10.1016/j.addr.2010.02.004

[12] Kim, C-j, *Natural polymers and their modification: Chitosan*, in *Advanced Pharmaceutics: Physicochemical Principles*. 2004, CRC Press. p 484-486.

[13] Domard, A and Rinaudo, M. Preparation and characterization of fully deacetylated chitosan. *International Journal of Biological Macromolecules,* 1983, 5, 49-51.

[14] Senel, S and McClure, SJ. Potential applications of chitosan in veterinary medicine. *Advanced Drug Delivery Reviews*, 2004, 56, 1467-1480.

[15] Lehr, CM; Bouwstra, JA; Schacht, EH and Junginger, HE. Invitro Evaluation of Mucoadhesive Properties of Chitosan and Some Other Natural Polymers. *International Journal of Pharmaceutics*, 1992, 78, 43-48.

[16] He, P; Davis, SS and Illum, L. In vitro evaluation of the mucoadhesive properties of chitosan microspheres. *International Journal of Pharmaceutics*, 1998, 166, 75-88.

[17] Miyazaki, S; Nakayama, A; Oda, M; Takada, M and Attwood, D. Chitosan and Sodium Alginate Based Bioadhesive Tablets for Intraoral Drug-Delivery. *Biological and Pharmaceutical Bulletin*, 1994, 17, 745-747.

[18] Genta, I; Conti, B; Perugini, P; Pavanetto, F; Spadaro, A and Puglisi, G. Bioadhesive microspheres for ophthalmic administration of acyclovir. *Journal of Pharmacy and Pharmacology*, 1997, 49, 737-742.

[19] Genta, I; Costantini, M and Montanari, L. Chitosan microspheres for nasal delivery: Effect of cross-linking agents on release characteristics. *23rd International Symposium on Controlled Release of Bioactive Materials, 1996 Proceedings*, 1996, 377-378

[20] Jameela, SR; Kumary, TV; Lal, AV and Jayakrishnan, A. Progesterone-loaded chitosan microspheres: a long acting biodegradable controlled delivery system. *Journal of Controlled Release*, 1998, 52, 17-24.

[21] Lefler, A and Ghanem, A. Development of bFGF-chitosan matrices and their interactions with human dermal fibroblast cells. *Journal of Biomaterials Science, Polymer Edition*, 2009, 20, 1335-1351.

[22] Azad, AK; Sermsintham, N; Chandrkrachang, S and Stevens, WF. Chitosan membrane as a wound-healing dressing: Characterization and clinical application. *Journal of Biomedical Materials Research Part B-Applied Biomaterials*, 2004, 69B, 216-222.

[23] Amidi, M; Mastrobattista, E; Jiskoot, W and Hennink, WE. Chitosan-based delivery systems for protein therapeutics and antigens. *Advanced Drug Delivery Reviews*, 2009, 62, 59-82.

[24] Gao, S; Chen, J; Xu, X; Ding, Z; Yang, Y-H; Hua, Z and Zhang, J. Galactosylated low molecular weight chitosan as DNA carrier for hepatocyte-targeting. *International Journal of Pharmaceutics*, 2003, 255, 57-68.

[25] Singla, AK and Chawla, M. Chitosan: some pharmaceutical and biological aspects - an update. *Journal of Pharmacy and Pharmacology*, 2001, 53, 1047-1067.

[26] Issa, MM; Köping-Höggård, M; Tømmeraas, K; Vårum, KM; Christensen, BE; Strand, SP and Artursson, P. Targeted gene delivery with trisaccharide-substituted chitosan oligomers in vitro and after lung administration in vivo. *Journal of Controlled Release*, 2006, 115, 103-112.

[27] Errington, N; Harding, SE; Vårum, KM and Illum, L. Hydrodynamic characterization of chitosans varying in degree of acetylation. *International Journal of Biological Macromolecules*, 1993, 15, 113-117.

[28] Soane, RJ; Frier, M; Perkins, AC; Jones, NS; Davis, SS and Illum, L. Evaluation of the clearance characteristics of bioadhesive systems in humans. *International Journal of Pharmaceutics*, 1999, 178, 55-65.

[29] Bhattarai, N; Gunn, J and Zhang, M. Chitosan-based hydrogels for controlled, localized drug delivery. *Advanced Drug Delivery Reviews*, 2009, 62, 83-99.

[30] Maillard-Salin, DG; Bécourt, P and Couarraze, G. A study of the adhesive-skin interface: correlation between adhesion and passage of a drug. *International Journal of Pharmaceutics*, 2000, 200, 121-126.

[31] Gao, S and Singh, J. In vitro percutaneous absorption enhancement of a lipophilic drug tamoxifen by terpenes. *Journal of Controlled Release*, 1998, 51, 193-199.

[32] Madgulkar, A; Kadam, S and Pokharkar, V. Studies on formulation development of mucoadhesive sustained release itraconazole tablet using response rurface methodology. *AAPS PharmSciTech*, 2008, 9, 998-1005.

[33] Park, H. and Robinson, JR. Mechanisms of mucoadhesion of poly(acrylic acid) hydrogels, *Pharmaceutical Research,* 1987, 4, 457-464.

[34] Tur, KM and Ch'ng, HS. Evaluation of possible mechanism(s) of bioadhesion. *International Journal of Pharmaceutics*, 1998, 160, 61-74.

[35] Smith, JM; Dornish, M and Wood, EJ. Involvement of protein kinase C in chitosan glutamate-mediated tight junction disruption. *Biomaterials*, 2005, 26, 3269-3276.

[36] Dodane, V; Amin Khan, M and Merwin, JR. Effect of chitosan on epithelial permeability and structure. *International Journal of Pharmaceutics*, 1999, 182, 21-32.

[37] Valenta, C and Auner, BG. The use of polymers for dermal and transdermal delivery. *European Journal of Pharmaceutics and Biopharmaceutics*, 2004, 58, 279-289.

[38] Sandri, G; Rossi, S; Bonferoni, MC; Ferrari, F; Zambito, Y; Di Colo, G and Caramella, C. Influence of n-trimethylation degree on buccal penetration enhancement properties of n-trimethyl chitosan: absorption of a high molecular weight molecule. *European Journal of Pharmaceutical Sciences*, 2005, 25, 8-10.

[39] Chiellini, F; Piras, AM; Errico, C and Chiellini, E. Micro/nanostructured polymeric systems for biomedical and pharmaceutical applications. *Nanomedicine*, 2008, 3, 367-393.

[40] Nicol, S. Life after Death for Empty Shells. *New Scientist*, 1991, 129, 46-48.

[41] Li, Q; Grandmaison, EW; Goosen, MFA and Dunn, ET. Applications and properties of chitosan. *Journal of Bioactive and Compatible Polymers*, 1992, 7, 370-397.

[42] Sezer, AD; Cevher, E; Hatipoglu, F; Ogurtan, Z; Bas, AL and Akbuga, J. The use of fucosphere in the treatment of dermal burns in rabbits. *European Journal of Pharmaceutics and Biopharmaceutics*, 2008, 69, 189-198.

[43] Ueno, H; Mori, T and Fujinaga, T. Topical formulations and wound healing applications of chitosan. *Advanced Drug Delivery Reviews*, 2001, 52, 105-115.

[44] Francis Suh, JK and Matthew, HWT. Application of chitosan-based polysaccharide biomaterials in cartilage tissue engineering: a review. *Biomaterials*, 2000, 21, 2589-2598.

[45] Yamane, S; Iwasaki, N; Majima, T; Funakoshi, T; Masuko, T; Harada, K; Minami, A; Monde, K and Nishimura, S-i. Feasibility of chitosan-

based hyaluronic acid hybrid biomaterial for a novel scaffold in cartilage tissue engineering. *Biomaterials*, 2005, 26, 611-619.

[46] Jeon, YJ; Park, PJ and Kim, SK. Antimicrobial effect of chitooligosaccharides produced by bioreactor. *Carbohydrate Polymers*, 2001, 44, 71-76.

[47] No, HK; Young Park, N; Ho Lee, S and Meyers, SP. Antibacterial activity of chitosans and chitosan oligomers with different molecular weights. *International Journal of Food Microbiology*, 2002, 74, 65-72.

[48] Berger, J; Reist, M; Mayer, JM; Felt, O and Gurny, R. Structure and interactions in chitosan hydrogels formed by complexation or aggregation for biomedical applications. *European Journal of Pharmaceutics and Biopharmaceutics*, 2004, 57, 35-52.

[49] Peppas, NA, *Preface: Hydrogels in medicine and pharmacy*, in *Fundamentals*, N.A.

[50] Ofner, CM and M., K-GC, *Gels*, in *Encyclopedia of Pharmaceutical Technology*, J. Swarbrick, Editor. 2007, Informa Healthcare: New York, USA. p 1875-1891.

[51] Felt, O; Buri, P and Gurny, R. Chitosan: A unique polysaccharide for drug delivery. *Drug Development and Industrial Pharmacy*, 1998, 24, 979-993.

[52] Illum, L. Chitosan and its use as a pharmaceutical excipient. *Pharmaceutical Research*, 1998, 15, 1326-1331.

[53] Bae, YH and Kim, SW. Hydrogel delivery systems based on polymer blends, block co-polymers or interpenetrating networks. *Advanced Drug Delivery Reviews*, 1993, 11, 109-135.

[54] Hamidi, M; Azadi, A and Rafiei, P. Hydrogel nanoparticles in drug delivery. *Advanced Drug Delivery Reviews*, 2008, 60, 1638-1649.

[55] Hennink, WE and van Nostrum, CF. Novel crosslinking methods to design hydrogels. *Advanced Drug Delivery Reviews*, 2002, 54, 13-36.

[56] Rinaudo, M. Chitin and chitosan: Properties and applications. *Progress in Polymer Science*, 2006, 31, 603-632.

[57] Ballantyne, B and Myers, RC. The acute toxicity and primary irritancy of glutaraldehyde solutions. *Veterinary and Human Toxicology*, 2001, 43, 193-202.

[58] Mi, F-L; Tan, Y-C; Liang, H-F and Sung, H-W. In vivo biocompatibility and degradability of a novel injectable-chitosan-based implant. *Biomaterials*, 2002, 23, 181-191.

[59] Shu, XZ; Zhu, KJ and Song, WH. Novel pH-sensitive citrate cross-linked chitosan film for drug controlled release. *International Journal of Pharmaceutics*, 2001, 212, 19-28.

[60] Shu, XZ and Zhu, KJ. Controlled drug release properties of ionically cross-linked chitosan beads: the influence of anion structure. *International Journal of Pharmaceutics*, 2002, 233, 217-225.

[61] Draget, KI; Värum, KM; Moen, E; Gynnild, H and Smidsrød, O. Chitosan cross-linked with Mo(VI) polyoxyanions: A new gelling system. *Biomaterials*, 1992, 13, 635-638.

[62] Mi, F-L; Peng, C-K; Huang, M-F; Lo, S-H and Yang, C-C. Preparation and characterization of N-acetylchitosan, N-propionylchitosan and N-butyrylchitosan microspheres for controlled release of 6-mercaptourine. *Carbohydrate Polymers*, 2005, 60, 219-227.

[63] Kean, T and Thanou, M. Biodegradation, biodistribution and toxicity of chitosan. *Advanced Drug Delivery Reviews*, 62, 3-11.

[64] Bernkop-Schnürch, A; Humenberger, C and Valenta, C. Basic studies on bioadhesive delivery systems for peptide and protein drugs. *International Journal of Pharmaceutics*, 1998, 165, 217-225.

[65] Tsai, CJ; Hsu, LR; Fang, JY and Lin, HH. Chitosan hydrogel as a base for transdermal delivery of berberine and its evaluation in rat skin. *Biological and Pharmaceutical Bulletin*, 1999, 22, 397-401.

[66] Ozsoy, Y; Gungor, S and Cevher, E. Vehicle effects on in vitro release of tiaprofenic acid from different topical formulations. *Il Farmaco*, 2004, 59, 563-566.

[67] Ozcan, I; Abaci, O; Haliki Uztan, A; Aksu, B; Boyacioglu, H; Guneri, T; Ozer, O. Enhanced topical delivery of terbinafine hydrochloride with chitosan hydrogels. *AAPS PharmSciTech,* 2009, 10, 1024-1031.

[68] Fang, JY; Leu, YL; Wang, YY and Tsai, YH. In vitro topical application and in vivo pharmacodynamic evaluation of nonivamide hydrogels using Wistar rat as an animal model. *European Journal of Pharmaceutical Sciences*, 2002, 15, 417-423.

[69] Cerchiara, T; Luppi, B; Chidichimo, G; Bigucci, F and Zecchi, V. Chitosan and poly(methyl vinyl ether-co-maleic anhydride) microparticles as nasal sustained delivery systems. *European Journal of Pharmaceutics and Biopharmaceutics*, 2005, 61, 195-200.

[70] Senyigit, T; Padula, C; Ozer, O and Santi, P. Different approaches for improving skin accumulation of topical corticosteroids. *International Journal of Pharmaceutics*, 2009, 380, 155-160.

[71] Ramanathan, S and Block, LH. The use of chitosan gels as matrices for electrically-modulated drug delivery. *Journal of Controlled Release*, 2001, 70, 109-123.

[72] Taveira, SF; Nomizo, A and Lopez, RFV. Effect of the iontophoresis of a chitosan gel on doxorubicin skin penetration and cytotoxicity. *Journal of Controlled Release*, 2009, 134, 35-40.

[73] Kumar, MNVR. A review of chitin and chitosan applications. *Reactive and Functional Polymers*, 2000, 46, 1-27.

[74] Obara, K; Ishihara, M; Ishizuka, T; Fujita, M; Ozeki, Y; Maehara, T; Saito, Y; Yura, H; Matsui, T; Hattori, H; Kikuchi, M and Kurita, A. Photocrosslinkable chitosan hydrogel containing fibroblast growth factor-2 stimulates wound healing in healing-impaired db/db mice. *Biomaterials*, 2003, 24, 3437-3444.

[75] He, W; Guo, X and Zhang, M. Transdermal permeation enhancement of N-trimethyl chitosan for testosterone. *International Journal of Pharmaceutics*, 2008, 356, 82-87.

[76] Padula, C; Nicoli, S and Santi, P. Innovative formulations for the delivery of levothyroxine to the skin. *International Journal of Pharmaceutics*, 2009, 372, 12-16.

[77] Modrzejewska, Z and Eckstein, W. Chitosan hollow fiber membranes. *Biopolymers*, 2004, 73, 61-68.

[78] Kam, HM; Khor, E and Lim, LY. Storage of partially deacetylated chitosan films. *J Biomed Mater Res*, 1999, 48, 881-888.

[79] Khan, TA; Peh K. K. and S., CnH. Mechanical, Bioadhesive strength and biological evaluations of chitosan films for wound dressing. *J Pharm Pharmaceut Sci*, 2000, 3, 303-311.

[80] Kim, E-M; Jeong, H-J; Kim, S-L; Sohn, M-H; Nah, J-W; Bom, H-S; Park, I-K and Cho, C-S. Asialoglycoprotein-receptor-targeted hepatocyte imaging using ^{99m}Tc galactosylated chitosan. *Nuclear Medicine and Biology*, 2006, 33, 529-534.

[81] Larena, A and Caceres, DA. Variability between chitosan membrane surface characteristics as function of its composition and environmental conditions. *Applied Surface Science*, 2004, 238, 273-277.

[82] Yan, X-L; Khor, E and Lim, LY. Chitosan-alginate films prepared with chitosans of different molecular weights. *Journal of Biomedical Materials Research*, 2000, 58,353-365.

[83] Thein-Han, WW and Stevens, WF. Transdermal delivery controlled by a chitosan membrane. *Drug Development and Industrial Pharmacy*, 2004, 30, 397-404.

[84] Chatelet, C; Damour, O and Domard, A. Influence of the degree of acetylation on some biological properties of chitosan films. *Biomaterials*, 2001, 22, 261-268.

[85] Mi, FL; Wu, YB; Shyu, SS; Chao, AC; Lai, JY and Su, CC. Asymmetric chitosan membranes prepared by dry/wet phase separation: a new type of wound dressing for controlled antibacterial release. *Journal of Membrane Science*, 2003, 212, 237-254.

[86] Silva, CL; Pereira, JC; Ramalho, A; Pais, AACC and Sousa, JJS. Films based on chitosan polyelectrolyte complexes for skin drug delivery: Development and characterization. *Journal of Membrane Science*, 2008, 320, 268-279.

[87] Wahid, A; Sridhar, BK and Shivakumar, S. Preparation and evaluation of transdermal drug delivery system of etoricoxib using modified chitosan. *Indian Journal of Pharmaceutical Science*, 2008, 70, 455-460.

[88] Thacharodi, D and Rao, KP. Release of nifedipine through cross-linked chitosan membranes. *International Journal of Pharmaceutics*, 1993, 96, 33-39.

[89] Dhanikula, AB and Panchagnula, R. Development and characterization of biodegradable chitosan films for local delivery of paclitaxel. *AAPS Journal*, 2004, 6, 88-99.

[90] Choi, YS; Lee, SB; Hong, SR; Lee, YM; Song, KW and Park, MH. Studies on gelatin-based sponges. Part III: a comparative study of cross-linked gelatin/alginate, gelatin/hyaluronate and chitosan/hyaluronate sponges and their application as a wound dressing in full-thickness skin defect of rat. *Journal of Materials Science: Materials in Medicine,* 2001, 12, 67-73.

[91] Kofuji, K; Qian, C-J; Nishimura, M; Sugiyama, I; Murata, Y and Kawashima, S. Relationship between physicochemical characteristics and functional properties of chitosan. *European Polymer Journal*, 2005, 41, 2784-2791.

[92] Mi, F-L; Shyu, S-S; Wu, Y-B; Lee, S-T; Shyong, J-Y and Huang, R-N. Fabrication and characterization of a sponge-like asymmetric chitosan membrane as a wound dressing. *Biomaterials*, 2001, 22, 165-173.

[93] Lai, HL; Abu'Khalil, A and Craig, DQM. The preparation and characterisation of drug-loaded alginate and chitosan sponges. *International Journal of Pharmaceutics*, 2003, 251, 175-181.

[94] Dai, M; Zheng, XL; Xu, X; Kong, XY; Li, XY; Guo, G; Luo, F; Zhao, X; Wei, YQ and Qian, ZY. Chitosan-alginate sponge: Preparation and application in curcumin delivery for dermal wound healing in rat.

Journal   of   Biomedicine   and   Biotechnology,   2009,
doi:10.1155/2009/595126.

[95] Denkbas, EB; Ozturk, E; Ozdemir, N; Kececi, K and Agalar, C.
Norfloxacin-loaded chitosan sponges as wound dressing material.
Journal of Biomaterials Applications, 2004, 18, 291-303.

[96] Wang, W; Lin, S; Xiao, Y; Huang, Y; Tan, Y; Cai, L and Li, X.
Acceleration of diabetic wound healing with chitosan-crosslinked
collagen sponge containing recombinant human acidic fibroblast growth
factor in healing-impaired STZ diabetic rats. *Life Science,* 2008, 82,
190-204.

[97] Moshfeghi, AA and Peyman, GA. Micro- and nanoparticulates.
Advanced Drug Delivery Reviews, 2005, 57, 2047-2052.

[98] Werle, M and Bernkop-Schnurch, A. Thiolated chitosans: useful
excipients for oral drug delivery. *Journal of Pharmacy and
Pharmacology,* 2008, 60, 273-281.

[99] Yang, M; Velaga, S; Yamamoto, H; Takeuchi, H; Kawashima, Y;
Hovgaard, L; van de Weert, M and Frokjaer, S. Characterisation of
salmon calcitonin in spray-dried powder for inhalation - Effect of
chitosan. *International Journal of Pharmaceutics,* 2007, 331, 176-181.

[100] Lim, ST; Martin, GP; Berry, DJ and Brown, MB. Preparation and
evaluation of the in vitro drug release properties and mucoadhesion of
novel microspheres of hyaluronic acid and chitosan. *Journal of
Controlled Release,* 2000, 66, 281-292.

[101] Agrawal, P; Strijkers, GJ and Nicolay, K. Chitosan-based systems for
molecular imaging. *Advanced Drug Delivery Reviews,* 2009, 62, 42-58.

[102] Pavanetto, F; Perugini, P; Conti, B; Modena, T and Genta, I. Evaluation
of process parameters involved in chitosan microsphere preparation by
the o/w/o multiple emulsion method. *Journal of Microencapsulation,*
1996, 13, 679-688.

[103] Orienti, I; Aiedeh, K; Gianasi, E; Bertasi, V and Zecchi, V.
Indomethacin loaded chitosan microspheres. Correlation between the
erosion process and release kinetics. *Journal of Microencapsulation,*
1996, 13, 463-472.

[104] Ohya, Y; Takei, T; Kobayashi, H and Ouchi, T. Release behavior of 5-
fluorouracil from chitosan-gel microspheres immobilizing 5-fluorouracil
derivative coated with polysaccharides and their cell specific
recognition. *Journal of Microencapsulation,* 1993, 10, 1-9.

[105] Calvo, P; RemunanLopez, C; VilaJato, JL and Alonso, MJ. Chitosan and
chitosan ethylene oxide propylene oxide block copolymer nanoparticles

as novel carriers for proteins and vaccines. *Pharmaceutical Research*, 1997, 14, 1431-1436.

[106] Sezer, AD; Cevher, E; Hatipoglu, F; Ogurtan, Z; Bas, AL and Akbuga, J. Preparation of Fucoidan-Chitosan Hydrogel and Its Application as Burn Healing Accelerator on Rabbits. *Biological and Pharmaceutical Bulletin*, 2008, 31, 2326-2333.

[107] Wan, LSC; Lim, LY and Soh, BL. Drug-Release from Chitosan Beads. *STP Pharma Sciences*, 1994, 4, 195-200.

[108] Hassan, EE; Parish, RC and Gallo, JM. Optimized formulation of magnetic chitosan microspheres containing the anticancer agent, oxantrazole. *Pharmaceutical Research*, 1992, 9, 390-397.

[109] Altaf, MA; Sreedharan and Charyulu, N. Ionic gelation controlled drug delivery systems for gastric-mucoadhesive microcapsules of captopril. *Indian Journal of Pharmaceutical Sciences*, 2008, 70, 655-658.

[110] Jain, SK; Chourasia, MK; Sabitha, M; Jain, R; Jain, AK; Ashawat, M and Jha, AK. Development and characterization of transdermal drug delivery systems for diltiazem hydrochloride. *Drug Delivery*, 2003, 10, 169-177.

[111] Nishioka, Y; Kyotani, S; Okamura, M; Miyazaki, M; Okazaki, K; Ohnishi, S; Yamamoto, Y and Ito, K. Release characteristics of cisplatin chitosan microspheres and effect of containing chitin. *Chemical and Pharmaceutical Bulletin*, 1990, 38, 2871-2873.

[112] Jameela, SR; Latha, PG; Subramoniam, A and Jayakrishnan, A. Antitumour activity of mitoxantrone-loaded chitosan microspheres against Ehrlich ascites carcinoma. *Journal of Pharmacy and Pharmacology*, 1996, 48, 685-688.

[113] Singh, UV and Udupa, N. Methotrexate loaded chitosan and chitin microspheres - in vitro characterization and pharmacokinetics in mice bearing Ehrlich ascites carcinoma. *J Microencapsul*, 1998, 15, 581-594.

[114] Chandy, T; Rao, GHR; Wilson, RF and Das, GS. Development of poly(lactic acid)/chitosan co-matrix microspheres: Controlled release of taxol-heparin for preventing restenosis. *Drug Delivery*, 2001, 8, 77-86.

[115] Kumbar, SG; Kulkarni, AR and Aminabhavi, TM. Crosslinked chitosan microspheres for encapsulation of diclofenac sodium: effect of crosslinking agent. *Journal of Microencapsulation*, 2002, 19, 173-180.

[116] Berthold, A; Cremer, K and Kreuter, J. Preparation and characterization of chitosan microspheres as drug carrier for prednisolone sodium phosphate as model for antiinflammatory drugs. *Journal of Controlled Release*, 1996, 39, 17-25.

[117] Genta, I; Pavanetto, F; Conti, B; Giunchedi, P and Conte, U. Improvement of Dexamethasone Dissolution Rate from Spray-Dried Chitosan Microspheres. *STP Pharma Sciences*, 1995, 5, 202-207.

[118] Bodmeier, R; Oh, KH and Pramar, Y. Preparation and evaluation of drug-containing chitosan beads. *Drug Development and Industrial Pharmacy*, 1989, 15, 1475-1494.

[119] Kulkarni, PV; Keshavayya, J and Kulkarni, VH. Effect of method of preparation and process variables on controlled release of insoluble drug from chitosan microspheres. *Polymers for Advanced Technologies*, 2007, 18, 814-821.

[120] Varshosaz, J; Dehkordi, AJ and Golafshan, S. Colon-specific delivery of mesalazine chitosan microspheres. *Jornal of Microencapsulation*, 2006, 23, 329-339.

[121] Kang, ML; Jiang, HL; Kang, SG; Guo, DD; Lee, DY; Cho, CS and Yoo, HS. Pluronic((R)) F127 enhances the effect as an adjuvant of chitosan microspheres in the intranasal delivery of Bordetella bronchiseptica antigens containing dermonecrotoxin. *Vaccine*, 2007, 25, 4602-4610.

[122] Huang, L; Xin, JY; Guo, YC and Li, JS. A Novel Insulin oral delivery system assisted by cationic beta-cyclodextrin polymers. *Journal of Applied Polymer Science*, 2010, 115, 1371-1379.

[123] Lee, JE; Kim, KE; Kwon, IC; Ahn, HJ; Lee, SH; Cho, HC; Kim, HJ; Seong, SC and Lee, MC. Effects of the controlled-released TGF-beta 1 from chitosan microspheres on chondrocytes cultured in a collagen/chitosan/glycosaminoglycan scaffold. *Biomaterials*, 2004, 25, 4163-4173.

[124] Akbuga, J; Ozbas-Turan, S and Erdogan, N. Plasmid-DNA loaded chitosan microspheres for in vitro IL-2 expression. *European Journal of Pharmaceutics and Biopharmaceutics*, 2004, 58, 501-507.

[125] Borchard, G. Chitosans for gene delivery. *Advanced Drug Delivery Reviews*, 2001, 52, 145-150.

[126] Remunan-Lopez, C; Portero, A; Lemos, M; Vila-Jato, JL; Nunez, MJ; Riveiro, P; Lopez, JM; Piso, M and Alonso, MJ. Chitosan microspheres for the specific delivery of amoxycillin to the gastric cavity. *STP Pharma Sciences*, 2000, 10, 69-76.

[127] Hejazi, R and Amiji, M. Stomach-specific anti-H-pylori therapy. II. Gastric residence studies of tetracycline-loaded chitosan microspheres in gerbils. *Pharmaceutical Development and Technology*, 2003, 8, 253-262.

[128] Giunchedi, P; Genta, I; Conti, B; Muzzarelli, RAA and Conte, U. Preparation and characterization of ampicillin loaded methylpyrrolidinone chitosan and chitosan microspheres. *Biomaterials*, 1998, 19, 157-161.

[129] Dhawan, S; Singla, AS and Sinha, VR. Evaluation of mucoadhesive properties of chitosan microspheres prepared by different dethods. *AAPS PharmSciTech*, 2004, 5, 1-7.

[130] Conti, B; Giunchedi, P; Genta, I and Conte, U. The preparation and in vivo evaluation of the wound-healing properties of chitosan microspheres. *STP Pharma Sciences*, 2000, 10, 101-104.

[131] Liu, H; Fan, H; Cui, Y; Chen, Y; Yao, K and Goh, JC. Effects of the controlled-released basic fibroblast growth factor from chitosan-gelatin microspheres on human fibroblasts cultured on a chitosan-gelatin scaffold. *Biomacromolecules*, 2007, 8, 1446-1455.

[132] Pitaksuteepong, T; Somsiri, A and Waranuch, N. Targeted transfollicular delivery of artocarpin extract from Artocarpus incisus by means of microparticles. *European Journal of Pharmaceutics and Biopharmaceutics*, 2007, 67, 639-645.

[133] Lira, AA; Rossetti, FC; Nanclares, DM; Neto, AF; Bentley, MV and Marchetti, JM. Preparation and characterization of chitosan-treated alginate microparticles incorporating all-trans retinoic acid. *Journal of Microencapsulation*, 2008, 26, 243-250.

[134] Alvarez-Román, R; Naik, A; Kalia, YN; Guy, RH and Fessi, H. Skin penetration and distribution of polymeric nanoparticles. *Journal of Controlled Release*, 2004, 99, 53-62.

[135] Maia, CS; Mehnert, W; Schaller, M; Korting, HC; Gysler, A; Haberland, A and Schafer-Korting, M. Drug targeting by solid lipid nanoparticles for dermal use. *Journal of Drug Targeting*, 2002, 10, 489-495.

[136] Katas, H and Alpar, HO. Development and characterisation of chitosan nanoparticles for siRNA delivery. *Journal of Controlled Release*, 2006, 115, 216-225.

[137] Senyigit, T; Sonvico, F; Barbieri, S; Ozer, O; Santi, P and Colombo, P. Lecithin/chitosan nanoparticles of clobetasol-17-propionate capable of accumulation in pig skin. *Journal of Controlled Release*, 2010, 142, 368-373.

[138] Mao, HQ; Roy, K; Troung-Le, VL; Janes, KA; Lin, KY; Wang, Y; August, JT and Leong, KW. Chitosan-DNA nanoparticles as gene carriers: synthesis, characterization and transfection efficiency. *Journal of Controlled Release*, 2001, 70, 399-421.

[139] Grenha, A; Seijo, B; Serra, C and Remunan-Lopez, C. Chitosan nanoparticle-loaded mannitol microspheres: Structure and surface characterization. *Biomacromolecules*, 2007, 8, 2072-2079.

[140] Tokumitsu, H; Ichikawa, H; Fukumori, Y and Block, LH. Preparation of gadopentetic acid-loaded chitosan microparticles for gadolinium neutron-capture therapy of cancer by a novel emulsion-droplet coalescence technique. *Chemical and Pharmaceutical Bulletin*, 1999, 47, 838-842.

[141] Fernandez-Urrusuno, R; Calvo, P; Remunan-Lopez, C; Vila-Jato, JL and Alonso, MJ. Enhancement of nasal absorption of insulin using chitosan nanoparticles. *Pharmaceutical Research*, 1999, 16, 1576-1581.

[142] Mitra, S; Gaur, U; Ghosh, PC and Maitra, AN. Tumour targeted delivery of encapsulated dextran-doxorubicin conjugate using chitosan nanoparticles as carrier. *Journal of Controlled Release*, 2001, 74, 317-323.

[143] Sinha, VR; Singla, AK; Wadhawan, S; Kaushik, R; Kumria, R; Bansal, K and Dhawan, S. Chitosan microspheres as a potential carrier for drugs. *International Journal of Pharmaceutics*, 2004, 274, 1-33.

[144] Hasanovic, A; Zehl, M; Reznicek, G and Valenta, C. Chitosan-tripolyphosphate nanoparticles as a possible skin drug delivery system for aciclovir with enhanced stability. *Journal of Pharmacy and Pharmacology*, 2009, 61, 1609-1616.

[145] Kim, DG; Jeong, YI; Choi, C; Roh, SH; Kang, SK; Jang, MK and Nah, JW. Retinol-encapsulated low molecular water-soluble chitosan nanoparticles. *International Journal of Pharmaceutics*, 2006, 319, 130-138.

[146] Colonna, C; Conti, B; Perugini, P; Pavanetto, F; Modena, T; Dorati, R; Iadarola, P and Genta, I. Ex vivo evaluation of prolidase loaded chitosan nanoparticles for the enzyme replacement therapy. *European Journal of Pharmaceutics and Biopharmaceutics*, 2008, 70, 58-65.

[147] Bal, SM; Slütter, B; van Riet, E; Kruithof, AC; Ding, Z; Kersten, GFA; Jiskoot, W and Bouwstra, JA. Efficient induction of immune responses through intradermal vaccination with N-trimethyl chitosan containing antigen formulations. *Journal of Controlled Release*, 142, 374-383.

[148] Cui, ZR and Mumper, RJ. Chitosan-based nanoparticles for topical genetic immunization. *Journal of Controlled Release*, 2001, 75, 409-419.

[149] Lee, P-W; Peng, S-F; Su, C-J; Mi, F-L; Chen, H-L; Wei, M-C; Lin, H-J and Sung, H-W. The use of biodegradable polymeric nanoparticles in

combination with a low-pressure gene gun for transdermal DNA delivery. *Biomaterials*, 2008, 29, 742-751.

[150] Lee, PW; Hsu, SH; Tsai, JS; Chen, FR; Huang, PJ; Ke, CJ; Liao, ZX; Hsiao, CW; Lin, HJ and Sung, HW. Multifunctional core-shell polymeric nanoparticles for transdermal DNA delivery and epidermal Langerhans cells tracking. *Biomaterials*, 2010, 31, 2425-2434.

[151] Ozbas-Turan, S; Akbuga, J and Sezer, AD. Topical Application of Antisense Oligonucleotide-Loaded Chitosan Nanoparticles to Rats. *Oligonucleotides*. In press. doi: 10.1089/oli.2009.0222.

[152] Chung, TW; Yang, MC and Tsai, WJ. A fibrin encapsulated liposomes-in-chitosan matrix (FLCM) for delivering water-soluble drugs. Influences of the surface properties of liposomes and the crosslinked fibrin network. *International Journal of Pharmaceutics*, 2006, 311, 122-129.

[153] Volodkin, D; Mohwald, H; Voegel, JC and Ball, V. Coating of negatively charged liposomes by polylysine: drug release study. *Journal of Controlled Release*, 2007, 117, 111-120.

[154] Kirjavainen, M; Monkkonen, J; Saukkosaari, M; Valjakka-Koskela, R; Kiesvaara, J and Urtti, A. Phospholipids affect stratum corneum lipid bilayer fluidity and drug partitioning into the bilayers. *Journal of Controlled Release*, 1999, 58, 207-214.

[155] Foldvari, M; Gesztes, A and Mezei, M. Dermal drug delivery by liposome encapsulation: Clinical and electron microscopic studies. *Journal of Microencapsulation*, 1990, 7, 479-489.

[156] Valenta, C and Janisch, M. Permeation of cyproterone acetate through pig skin from different vehicles with phospholipids. *International Journal of Pharmaceutics*, 2003, 258, 133-139.

[157] Biruss, B and Valenta, C. Skin permeation of different steroid hormones from polymeric coated liposomal formulations. *European Journal of Pharmaceutics and Biopharmaceutics*, 2006, 62, 210-219.

[158] Mezei, M, *Liposome Technology- Interactions liposomes with the biological milieu*, in *Techniques for the study of liposome-skin interaction*, G. Gregoriadis, Editor. 1993, CRC Press, Inc.

[159] Foco, A; Gasperlin, M and Kristl, J. Investigation of liposomes as carriers of sodium ascorbyl phosphate for cutaneous photoprotection. *Int J Pharm*, 2005, 291,21-29.

[160] Shim, J; Kim, MJ; Kim, HK; Kim, DH; Oh, SG; Ko, SY; Jang, HG and Kim, JW. Morphological effect of lipid carriers on permeation of

lidocaine hydrochloride through lipid membranes. *International Journal of Pharmaceutics*, 2010, 388, 251-256.

[161] Perugini, P; Genta, I; Pavanetto, F; Conti, B; Scalia, S and Baruffini, A. Study on glycolic acid delivery by liposomes and microspheres. *International Journal of Pharmaceutics*, 2000, 196, 51-61.

[162] El Maghraby, GMM; Williams, AC and Barry, BW. Interactions of surfactants (edge activators) and skin penetration enhancers with liposomes. *International Journal of Pharmaceutics*, 2004, 276, 143-161.

[163] Walters, KA, *Drug Delivery: Topical and transdermal routes*, in *Encyclopedia of Pharmaceutical Technology*, J. Swarbrick, Editor. 2007, Informa Healthcare: North Carolinia, USA. p 1311-1325.

[164] Hasanovic, A; Hollick, C; Fischinger, K and Valenta, C. Improvement in physicochemical parameters of DPPC liposomes and increase in skin permeation of aciclovir and minoxidil by the addition of cationic polymers. *European Journal of Pharmaceutics and Biopharmaceutics*. In press. doi: 10.1016/j.ejpb.2010.03.014.

[165] Oku, N and Namba, Y. Long-circulating liposomes. *Critical Reviews in Therapeutic Drug Carrier Systems,* 1994, 11, 231-270.

[166] Thongborisute, J; Tsuruta, A; Kawabata, Y and Takeuchi, H. The effect of particle structure of chitosan-coated liposomes and type of chitosan on oral delivery of calcitonin. *Jornal of Drug Targeting*, 2006, 14, 147-154.

[167] Li, N; Zhuang, C; Wang, M; Sun, X; Nie, S and Pan, W. Liposome coated with low molecular weight chitosan and its potential use in ocular drug delivery. *International Journal of Pharmaceutics,* 2009, 379, 131-138.

[168] McPhail, D; Tetley, L; Dufes, C and Uchegbu, IF. Liposomes encapsulating polymeric chitosan based vesicles--a vesicle in vesicle system for drug delivery. *International Journal of Pharmaceutics,* 2000, 200, 73-86.

[169] Henriksen, I; Vagen, SR; Sande, SA; Smistad, G and Karlsen, J. Interactions between liposomes and chitosan II: effect of selected parameters on aggregation and leakage. *International Journal of Pharmaceutics*, 1997, 146, 193-204.

[170] Mady, MM; Darwish, MM; Khalil, S and Khalil, WM. Biophysical studies on chitosan-coated liposomes. *European Biophysics Journal*, 2009, 38, 1127-1133.

[171] Boulmedarat, L; Grossiord, JL; Fattal, E and Bochot, A. Influence of methyl-beta-cyclodextrin and liposomes on rheological properties of

Carbopol 974P NF gels. *International Journal of Pharmaceutics,* 2003, 254, 59-64.

[172] Alamelu, S and Rao, KP. Studies on the carboxymethyl chitosan-containing liposomes for their stability and controlled release of dapsone. *Journal of Microencapsulation,* 1991, 8, 505-519.

[173] Glavas-Dodov, M; Goracinova, K; Mladenovska, K and Fredro-Kumbaradzi, E. Release profile of lidocaine HCl from topical liposomal gel formulation. *International Journal of Pharmaceutics,* 2002, 242, 381-384.

[174] Glavas-Dodov, M; Fredro-Kumbaradzi, E; Goracinova, K; Calis, S; Simonoska, M and Hincal, AA. 5-Fluorouracil in topical liposome gels for anticancer treatment – Formulation and evaluation. *Acta Pharmaceutica,* 2003, 53, 241-150.

[175] Feng, SS; Ruan, G and Li, QT. Fabrication and characterizations of a novel drug delivery device liposomes-in-microsphere (LIM). *Biomaterials,* 2004, 25, 5181-5189.

[176] Gonzalez-Rodriguez, ML; Barros, LB; Palma, J; Gonzalez-Rodriguez, PL and Rabasco, AM. Application of statistical experimental design to study the formulation variables influencing the coating process of lidocaine liposomes. *International Journal of Pharmaceutics,* 2007, 337, 336-345.

[177] Takeuchi, H; Yamamoto, H; Niwa, T; Hino, T and Kawashima, Y. Enteral absorption of insulin in rats from mucoadhesive chitosan-coated liposomes. *Pharmaceutical Research,* 1996, 13, 896-901.

[178] Kozlova, NO; Bruskovskaya, IB; Melik-Nubarov, NS; Yaroslavov, AA and Kabanov, VA. Catalytic properties and conformation of hydrophobized alpha-chymotrypsin incorporated into a bilayer lipid membrane. *FEBS Letters,* 1999, 461, 141-144.

[179] Henriksen, I; Smistad, G and Karlsen, J. Interaction between liposomes and chitosan. *International Journal of Pharmaceutics,* 1994, 101, 227-236.

[180] Dong, C and Rogers, JA. Quantitative determination of carboxymethyl chitin in polymer-coated liposomes. *Journal of Microencapsulation,* 1991, 8, 153-160.

[181] Takeuchi, H; Matsui, Y; Yamamoto, H and Kawashima, Y. Mucoadhesive properties of carbopol or chitosan-coated liposomes and their effectiveness in the oral administration of calcitonin to rats. *Journal of Controlled Release,* 2003, 86, 235-242.

[182] Guo, P; Coban, O; Snead, N; Trebley, J; Hoeprich, S; Guo, S and Shu, Y. Engineering RNA for Targeted siRNA Delivery and Medical Application. *Advanced Drug Delivery Reviews*, In Press, doi: 10.1016/j.addr.2010.

[183] Galovic Rengel, R; Barisic, K; Pavelic, Z; Zanic Grubisic, T; Cepelak, I and Filipovic-Grcic, J. High efficiency entrapment of superoxide dismutase into mucoadhesive chitosan-coated liposomes. *European Journal of Pharmaceutical Science*, 2002, 15, 441-448.

[184] Ruel-Gariepy, E; Leclair, G; Hildgen, P; Gupta, A and Leroux, JC. Thermosensitive chitosan-based hydrogel containing liposomes for the delivery of hydrophilic molecules. *Journal of Controlled Release*, 2002, 82, 373-383.

[185] Biondi, M; Ungaro, F; Quaglia, F and Netti, PA. Controlled drug delivery in tissue engineering. *Advanced Drug Delivery Reviews*, 2008, 60, 229-242.

[186] Ng, KV; Khor, HL and Hutmacher, DW, *Biodegradable Systems in Tissue Engineering and Regenerative Medicine*, in *Skin Tissue Engineering Part II - The in vitro evaluation of natural and synthetic 3-D matrices as dermal substrates*, R.L. Reis and J.S. Roman, Editors. 2005, CRC Press.

[187] Naughton, G; Mansbridge, J and Gentzkow, G. A metabolically active human dermal replacement for the treatment of diabetic foot ulcers. *Artificial Organs*, 1997, 21, 1203-1210.

[188] Saintigny, G; Bonnard, M; Damour, O and Collombel, C. Reconstruction of epidermis on a chitosan cross-linked collagen-GAG lattice: effect of fibroblasts. *Acta Dermato Venereologica*, 1993, 73, 175-180.

[189] Lacroix, S; Bouez, C; Vidal, S; Cenizo, V; Reymermier, C; Justin, V; Vicanova, J and Damour, O. Supplementation with a complex of active nutrients improved dermal and epidermal characteristics in skin equivalents generated from fibroblasts from young or aged donors. *Biogerontology*, 2007, 8, 97-109.

[190] Dezutter-Dambuyant, C; Black, A; Bechetoille, N; Bouez, C; Marechal, S; Auxenfans, C; Cenizo, V; Pascal, P; Perrier, E and Damour, O. Evolutive skin reconstructions: from the dermal collagen-glycosaminoglycan-chitosane substrate to an immunocompetent reconstructed skin. *Biomedical Materials and Engineering*, 2006, 16, 85-94.

[191] Sokolsky-Papkov, M; Agashi, K; Olaye, A; Shakesheff, K and Domb, AJ. Polymer carriers for drug delivery in tissue engineering. *Advanced Drug Delivery Reviews*, 2007, 59, 187-206.

[192] Moharamzadeh, K; Brook, IM; Van Noort, R; Scutt, AM and Thornhill, MH. Tissue-engineered oral mucosa: a review of the scientific literature. *Journal of Dental Research*, 2007, 86, 115-124.

[193] Huang, S and Fu, X. Naturally derived materials-based cell and drug delivery systems in skin regeneration. *Journal of Controlled Release*, 2009, 142, 149-159.

[194] Ramshaw, JA; Mitrangas, K and Bateman, JF. Heterogeneity in dermatosparaxis is shown by contraction of collagen gels. *Connective Tissue Research*, 1991, 25, 295-300.

[195] Aoyagi, S; Onishi, H and Machida, Y. Novel chitosan wound dressing loaded with minocycline for the treatment of severe burn wounds. *International Journal of Pharmaceutics*, 2007, 330, 138-145.

[196] Adekogbe, I and Ghanem, A. Fabrication and characterization of DTBP-crosslinked chitosan scaffolds for skin tissue engineering. *Biomaterials*, 2005, 26, 7241-7250.

[197] Muzzarelli, RA; Mattioli-Belmonte, M; Pugnaloni, A and Biagini, G. Biochemistry, histology and clinical uses of chitins and chitosans in wound healing. *Exs*, 1999, 87, 251-264.

[198] Stone, CA; Wright, H; Clarke, T; Powell, R and Devaraj, VS. Healing at skin graft donor sites dressed with chitosan. *British Journal of Plastic Surgery*, 2000, 53, 601-606.

[199] Rossi, S; Marciello, M; Sandri, G; Ferrari, F; Bonferoni, MC; Papetti, A; Caramella, C; Dacarro, C and Grisoli, P. Wound dressings based on chitosans and hyaluronic acid for the release of chlorhexidine diacetate in skin ulcer therapy. *Pharmaceutical Development and Technology*, 2007, 12, 415-422.

[200] Boucard, N; Viton, C; Agay, D; Mari, E; Roger, T; Chancerelle, Y and Domard, A. The use of physical hydrogels of chitosan for skin regeneration following third-degree burns. *Biomaterials*, 2007, 28, 3478-3488.

[201] Ikemoto, S; Mochizuki, M; Yamada, M; Takeda, A; Uchinuma, E; Yamashina, S; Nomizu, M and Kadoya, Y. Laminin peptide-conjugated chitosan membrane: Application for keratinocyte delivery in wounded skin. *Journal of Biomedical Materials Research A*, 2006, 79, 716-722.

[202] Howling, GI; Dettmar, PW; Goddard, PA; Hampson, FC; Dornish, M and Wood, EJ. The effect of chitin and chitosan on the proliferation of

human skin fibroblasts and keratinocytes in vitro. *Biomaterials*, 2001, 22, 2959-2966.

[203] Li, QT; Dun, ET; Grandmaison, EW and Goosen, MFA, *Applications of Chitin and Chitosan*, in *Applications and properties of chitosan*, M.F.A. Goosen, Editor. 1997, CRC Press.

[204] Norazril, SA; Aminuddin, BS; Norhayati, MM; Mazlyzam, AL; Fauziah, O and Ruszymah, BH. Comparison of chitosan scaffold and chitosan-collagen scaffold: a preliminary study. *Medical Journal of Malaysia*, 2004, 59 Suppl B, 186-187.

[205] Ma, L; Gao, C; Mao, Z; Zhou, J; Shen, J; Hu, X and Han, C. Collagen/chitosan porous scaffolds with improved biostability for skin tissue engineering. *Biomaterials*, 2003, 24, 4833-4841.

[206] Shi, DH; Cai, DZ; Zhou, CR; Rong, LM; Wang, K and Xu, YC. Development and potential of biomimetic chitosan/ type II collagen scaffold for cartilage tissue engineering. *Chinese Mediacl Journal*, 2005, 118, 1436-1443.

[207] Elder, SH; Nettles, DL and Bumgardner, JD. Synthesis and characterization of chitosan scaffolds for cartilage-tissue engineering. *Methods in Molecular Biology*, 2004, 238, 41-48.

[208] Nastasescu, OS; Popa, IM; Verestiuc, L; Butnaru, M and Baran, D. Scaffolds based on collagen and chitosan for post-burn tissue engineering. *Revista Medico Chirurgicala a Societatii de Mededici si Naturalisti din Iasi*, 2008, 112, 547-553.

[209] Xu, SJ; Huang, AB; Ma, L; Teng, JY; Gao, CY; Zhang, ZL; Ni, YD; Ye, S and Wang, YG. Mechanisms and effects of biosynthesis and apoptosis in repair of full-thickness skin defect with collagen-chitosan dermal stent. *Zhonghua Zheng Xing Wai Ke Za Zhi*, 2009, 25, 208-212.

[210] Taravel, MN and Domard, A. Relation between the physicochemical characteristics of collagen and its interactions with chitosan: I. *Biomaterials*, 1993, 14, 930-938.

[211] Tangsadthakun, C; Kanokpanont, S; Sanchavanakit, N; Banaprasert, T and Damrongsakkul, S. Properties of collagen/chitosan scaffolds for skin tissue engineering. *Journal of Minerals, Metals and Materials,* 2006, 16, 37-44.

[212] Damour, O; Gueugniaud, PY; Berthin-Maghit, M; Rousselle, P; Berthod, F; Sahuc, F and Collombel, C. A dermal substrate made of collagen--GAG--chitosan for deep burn coverage: first clinical uses. *Clinical Materials*, 1994, 15, 273-276.

[213] Kellouche, S; Martin, C; Korb, G; Rezzonico, R; Bouard, D; Benbunan, M; Dubertret, L; Soler, C; Legrand, C and Dosquet, C. Tissue engineering for full-thickness burns: a dermal substitute from bench to bedside. *Biochemical Biophysical Reserach Communications*, 2007, 363, 472-478.

[214] Chen, KY; Liao, WJ; Kuo, SM; Tsai, FJ; Chen, YS; Huang, CY and Yao, CH. Asymmetric chitosan membrane containing collagen I nanospheres for skin tissue engineering. *Biomacromolecules*, 2009, 10, 1642-1649.

[215] Sun, LP; Wang, S; Zhang, ZW; Wang, XY and Zhang, QQ. Biological evaluation of collagen-chitosan scaffolds for dermis tissue engineering. *Biomedical Materials*, 2009, doi: 10.1088/1748-6041/4/5/055008.

[216] Mao, J; Zhao, L; De Yao, K; Shang, Q; Yang, G and Cao, Y. Study of novel chitosan-gelatin artificial skin in vitro. *Journal of Biomedical Materials Reserach A*, 2003, 64, 301-308.

[217] Yang, J; Yang, GH; Liu, W; Cui, L; Qian, YL and Cao, YL. Construction and clinical application of tissue engineered epidermal membrane. *Zhonghua Zheng Xing Wai Ke Za Zhi*, 2005, 21, 281-284.

[218] Park, CJ; Clark, SG; Lichtensteiger, CA; Jamison, RD and Johnson, AJ. Accelerated wound closure of pressure ulcers in aged mice by chitosan scaffolds with and without bFGF. *Acta Biomaterialia*, 2009, 5, 1926-1936.

[219] Liu, H; Mao, J; Yao, K; Yang, G; Cui, L and Cao, Y. A study on a chitosan-gelatin-hyaluronic acid scaffold as artificial skin in vitro and its tissue engineering applications. *Journal of Biomaterials Science Polymer Edition*, 2004, 15, 25-40.

[220] Liu, H; Yin, Y and Yao, K. Construction of chitosan-gelatin-hyaluronic acid artificial skin in vitro. *Journal of Biomaterials Applications*, 2007, 21, 413-430.

[221] Lim, CK; Yaacob, NS; Ismail, Z and Halim, AS. In vitro biocompatibility of chitosan porous skin regenerating templates (PSRTs) using primary human skin keratinocytes. *Toxicology In Vitro*, 2010, 24, 721-727.

[222] Niekraszewicz, A. Chitosan medical dressings. *Fibres Textiles*, 2005, 13, 16-18.

[223] Wanichwecharungruang, SP. Chitosan-nanoparticle as UV filter and carrier for cosmetic actives. *Nanotechnology*, 2007, 4, 257-260.

[224] Schlotmann, K; Kaeten, M; Black, AF; Damour, O; Waldmann-Laue, M and Forster, T. Cosmetic efficacy claims in vitro using a three-

dimensional human skin model. *International Journal of Cosmetic Science*, 2001, 23, 309-318.

[225] Anchisi, C; Meloni, MC and Maccioni, AM. Chitosan beads loaded with essential oils in cosmetic formulations. *International Journal of Cosmetic Science*, 2007, 29,485.

[226] Augustin, C; Frei, V; Perrier, E; Huc, A and Damour, O. A skin equivalent model for cosmetological trials: an in vitro efficacy study of a new biopeptide. *Skin Pharmacology*, 1997, 10, 63-70.

[227] Martini, MC and Seiller, M, eds. *Actifs et additifs en cosmetologie.* Chitosane, ed. C. Jacquot. Vol. 3. 2006, Lavoisier: Paris. p 315-334.

[228] Burkatovskaya, M; Castano, AP; Demidova-Rice, TN; Tegos, GP and Hamblin, MR. Effect of chitosan acetate bandage on wound healing in infected and noninfected wounds in mice. *Wound Repair and Regeneration*, 2008, 16, 425-431.

[229] Dai, T; Tegos, GP; Burkatovskaya, M; Castano, AP and Hamblin, MR. Chitosan acetate bandage as a topical antimicrobial dressing for infected burns. *Antimicrobial Agents and Chemotherapy*, 2009, 53, 393-400.

[230] Poretti, F; Rosen, T; Korner, B and Vorwerk, D. Chitosan pads vs. manual compression to control bleeding sites after transbrachial arterial catheterization in a randomized trial. *Fortschritte auf dem Gebiete der Röntgenstrahlen und der Nuklearmedizin,* 2005, 177, 1260-1266.

[231] Pillai, CKS; Paul, W and Sharma, CP. Chitin and chitosan polymers: Chemistry, solubility and fiber formation. *Progress in Polymer Science*, 2009, 34, 641-678.

[232] Yang, A and Wu, R. Mechanical properties and interfacial interaction of a novel bioabsorbable chitin fiber reinforced poly (ε-caprolactone) composite. *Journal of Materials Science Letters*, 2001, 20, 977-979.

[233] Yano, H; Iriyama, K; Nishiwaki, H and Kifune, K. Effect of Nacetyl- D-glucosamine on wound healing in rats. *Mie Medical Journal*, 1985, 35, 53-56.

[234] Benicewitz, BC and Hopper, PK. Polymers for absorbable surgical sutures. *Journal of Bioactive and Compatible Polymers*, 1991, 6, 64-94.

[235] Hu, W; Huang, ZM; Meng, SY and He, CL. Fabrication and characterization of chitosan coated braided PLLA wire using aligned electrospun fibers. *Journal of Materials Science: Materials in Medcicine*, 2009, 20, 2275-2284.

[236] Ito, Y; Hagiwara, E; Saeki, A; Sugioka, N and Takada, K. Feasibility of microneedles for percutaneous absorption of insulin. *European Journal of Pharmaceutical Science*, 2006, 29, 82-88.

[237] Ito, Y; Yoshimitsu, J; Shiroyama, K; Sugioka, N and Takada, K. Self-dissolving microneedles for the percutaneous absorption of EPO in mice. *Journal of Drug Targeting*, 2006, 14, 255-261.

[238] Xie, Y; Xu, B and Gao, Y. Controlled transdermal delivery of model drug compounds by MEMS microneedle array. *Nanomedicine*, 2005, 1, 184-190.

Index